COVID-19
Challenges Ahead

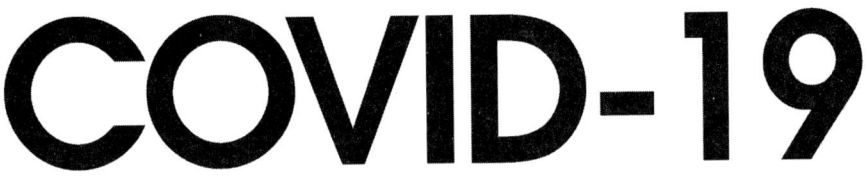

COVID-19
Challenges Ahead

Satyendra K Tiwary MBBS, MS, FICS, FMAS, FCLS
Associate Professor
Department of General Surgery
Institute of Medical Sciences
Banaras Hindu University, Varanasi
email: drsktiwary1@gmail.com, satyendrak.tiwary1@bhu.ac.in

Vishwambhar Singh MBBS, MS
Associate Professor
Department of Otorhinolaryngology
Institute of Medical Sciences
Banaras Hindu University, Varanasi
email: singhvishwambhar@gmail.com, singhvishwambhar@bhu.ac.in

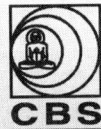

CBS

CBS Publishers & Distributors Pvt Ltd

New Delhi • Bengaluru • Chennai • Kochi • Kolkata • Mumbai
Hyderabad • Jharkhand • Nagpur • Patna • Pune • Uttarakhand

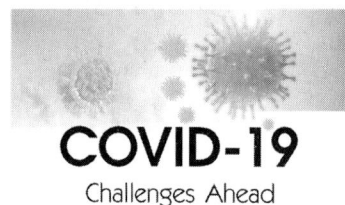

COVID-19
Challenges Ahead

ISBN: 978-93-88527-78-1

Copyright © Authors and Publisher

First Edition: 2020

Reprint: 2021

Published by Satish Kumar Jain and produced by Varun Jain for

CBS Publishers & Distributors Pvt Ltd
4819/XI Prahlad Street, 24 Ansari Road, Daryaganj, New Delhi 110 002, India.
Ph: 011-23289259, 23266861, 23266867 Fax: 011-23243014 Website: www.cbspd.com
e-mail: delhi@cbspd.com; cbspubs@airtelmail.in

Corporate Office: 204 FIE, Industrial Area, Patparganj, Delhi 110 092
Ph: 011-4934 4934   Fax: 011-4934 4935 e-mail: publishing@cbspd.com;publicity@cbspd.com

Branches

- **Bengaluru:** Seema House 2975, 17th Cross, K.R. Road,
  Banasankari 2nd Stage, Bengaluru 560 070, Karnataka
  Ph: +91-80-26771678/79   Fax: +91-80-26771680   e-mail: bangalore@cbspd.com
- **Chennai:** 7, Subbaraya Street, Shenoy Nagar, Chennai 600 030, Tamil Nadu
  Ph: +91-44-26680620, 26681266   Fax: +91-44-42032115   e-mail: chennai@cbspd.com
- **Kochi:** 42/1325, 1326, Power House Road, Opp KSEB, Power House,
  Ernakulam 682 018, Kerala, India
  Ph: +91-484-4059061-65   Fax: +91-484-4059065   e-mail: kochi@cbspd.com
- **Kolkata:** 6/B, Ground Floor, Rameswar Shaw Road, Kolkata-700 014, West Bengal
  Ph: +91-33-22891126, 22891127, 22891128   e-mail: kolkata@cbspd.com
- **Mumbai:** PWD Shed. Gala no. 25/26, Ramchandra Bhatt Marg, Next to JJ Hospital Gate no. 2,
  Opp. Union Bank of India, Noorbaug, Mumbai-400009, Maharashtra, India
  Ph: 022-66661880/89   e-mail: mumbai@cbspd.com

Representatives

• Hyderabad	0-9885175004	• Jharkhand	0-9811541605	• Nagpur	0-9421945513
• Patna	0-9334159340	• Pune	0-9623451994	• Uttarakhand	0-9716462459

Printed at Sanjay Printers, Patparganj Industrial Area, Delhi, India

Contributors

Abhishek Abhinay
Assistant Professor
Department of Paediatrics
Institute of Medical Sciences
Banaras Hindu University
Varanasi

Adity Prakash
Junior Resident
Department of Radiodiagnosis
Institute of Medical Sciences
Banaras Hindu University
Varanasi

Akhilesh Tiwari
Junior Resident
Department of TB and Respiratory Diseases
Institute of Medical Sciences
Banaras Hindu University
Varanasi

Amit Singh
Professor
Department of Pharmacology
Institute of Medical Sciences
Banaras Hindu University
Varanasi

Anish K Saha
Junior Resident
Department of General Medicine
Institute of Medical Sciences
Banaras Hindu University
Varanasi

Anjali Rani
Professor
Department of Obstetrics and Gynaecology
Institute of Medical Sciences
Banaras Hindu University
Varanasi

Arghya Das
Senior Resident
Department of Microbiology
Institute of Medical Sciences
Banaras Hindu University
Varanasi

Ashish Verma
Professor
Department of Radiodiagnosis
Institute of Medical Sciences
Banaras Hindu University
Varanasi

Ashvanee Kumar Chaudhary
Senior Resident
Department of ENT
Institute of Medical Sciences
Banaras Hindu University
Varanasi

Bhairav Pathak
Junior Resident
Department of Pharmacology
Institute of Medical Sciences
Banaras Hindu University
Varanasi

Bisweswar Ojha
Junior Resident
Department of Pharmacology
Institute of Medical Sciences
Banaras Hindu University
Varanasi

Deepak Kumar Gupta
Junior Resident
Department of ENT
Institute of Medical Sciences
Banaras Hindu University
Varanasi

Deepak K Gautam
Associate Professor
Department of General Medicine
Institute of Medical Sciences
Banaras Hindu University
Varanasi

Deepak Kumar Shah
Assistant Professor
Department of TB and Respiratory Diseases
Institute of Medical Sciences
Banaras Hindu University
Varanasi

Hemendra Singh
Senior Resident
Department of Ophthalmology
Institute of Medical Sciences
Banaras Hindu University
Varanasi

Ishan Kumar
Assistant Professor
Department of Radiodiagnosis
Institute of Medical Sciences
Banaras Hindu University
Varanasi

Kumar Sarvottam
Associate Professor
Department of Physiology
Institute of Medical Sciences
Banaras Hindu University
Varanasi

Mohit Mangla
Junior Resident
Department of General Surgery
Institute of Medical Sciences
Banaras Hindu University
Varanasi

Pallavi Gupta
Junior Resident
Department of Anaesthesiology and Critical Care
Institute of Medical Sciences
Banaras Hindu University
Varanasi

Pankaj Kumar Gupta
Assistant Professor
Department of Psychiatry
Institute of Medical Sciences
Banaras Hindu University
Varanasi

Prashant Bhusan
Associate Professor
Department of Ophthalmology
Institute of Medical Sciences
Banaras Hindu University
Varanasi

Raghunath S More
Associate Professor
Department of Anatomy
Institute of Medical Sciences
Banaras Hindu University
Varanasi

Rahul Garg
Senior Resident
Department of Microbiology
Institute of Medical Sciences
Banaras Hindu University
Varanasi

Rajeev Kumar Dubey
Professor
Department of Anaesthesiology and Critical Care
Institute of Medical Sciences
Banaras Hindu University
Varanasi

Rameshwar Nath Chaurasia
Professor and Head
Department of Neurology
Institute of Medical Sciences
Banaras Hindu University
Varanasi

Ruchi Birendra
Medical Officer Post-Partum
Department of Obstetrics and Gynaecology
Institute of Medical Sciences
Banaras Hindu University
Varanasi

SK Rao
Associate Professor
Department of Paediatrics
Institute of Medical Sciences
Banaras Hindu University
Varanasi

Sachchidanand
Assistant Professor
Community Medicine
Maharshi Vashishtha Autonomous
State Medical College
Basti, UP

Samir Kumar Singh
Assistant Professor
Department of Physiology
Institute of Medical Sciences
Banaras Hindu University
Varanasi

Satyendra K Tiwary
Associate Professor
Department of General Surgery
Institute of Medical Sciences
Banaras Hindu University
Varanasi

Sankha Shubhra Chakrabarti
Assistant Professor
Department of Geriatrics
Institute of Medical Sciences
Banaras Hindu University
Varanasi

Shikha Sachan
Associate Professor
Department of Obstetrics and Gynaecology
Institute of Medical Sciences
Banaras Hindu University
Varanasi

SP Mishra
Professor
Department of Biochemistry
Institute of Medical Sciences
Banaras Hindu University
Varanasi

Sunil Kumar
Associate Professor
Community Medicine
Institute of Medical Sciences
Banaras Hindu University
Varanasi

Tuhina Banerjee
Associate Professor
Department of Microbiology
Institute of Medical Sciences
Banaras Hindu University
Varanasi

Tulika Dey
Junior Research Fellow (UGC-CSIR)
Department of Biochemistry
Institute of Medical Sciences
Banaras Hindu University
Varanasi

Upinder Kaur
Assistant Professor
Department of Pharmacology
All India Institute of Medical Sciences
Gorakhpur

Varun Kumar Singh
Assistant Professor
Department of Neurology
Institute of Medical Sciences
Banaras Hindu University
Varanasi

Vishwambhar Singh
Associate Professor
Department of ENT
Institute of Medical Sciences
Banaras Hindu University
Varanasi

Foreword

History of human has been full with pages of struggles, innovations and challenges. COVID-19 in 2020 has metamorphosed the whole world in a drastic way leading to challenges in overall survival and global development. In this context, things are changing rapidly with addition of knowledge, protocol, and steps to safeguard the humankind. Best way to complete the task always requires input, analysis and conclusion. In this background, the team of authors from Institute of Medical Sciences, Banaras Hindu University has made an effort regarding updating and digitalizing the knowledge of COVID-19. Leading, coordinating and editing by Satyendra K Tiwary and Vishwambhar Singh has led this form of the book which will be very useful for gathering the knowledge about the COVID-19 from a single point source in a single book. In challenging times, contribution may be in many forms like donating, writing, encouraging and helping the needy ones. Academic inputs are important tools in such situation. Awareness, knowledge and coordination are essential at the time of crisis. Best efforts have been made by the team of doctors to bring the shape of this book.

I feel the task done by team bringing this book in present form is only one part of the whole efforts made so far in present time. Apart from academic activity, other much needed support to the society has been given by this team through various organisations such as National Medicos Organisation (NMO) and Seva Bharati which is a feather in the cap for all contributors in any form at this moment of crisis.

We will care, we will cure, we will conquer.

Finally, I close my words with the message from Kathopnishad:

उत्तिष्ठत जाग्रत प्राप्य वरान्निबोधत।

क्षुरस्य धारा निशिता दुरत्यया दुर्ग पथस्तत्कवयो वदन्ति।।

(कठोपनिषद्, अध्याय १, वल्ली ३, मंत्र १४)

(उत्तिष्ठत, जाग्रत, वरान् प्राप्य निबोधत। क्षुरस्य निशिता धारा (यथा) दुरत्यया (तथा एवआत्मज्ञानस्य) तत् पथः दुर्गं (इति) कवयः वदन्ति।)

जिसका अर्थ है: उठो, जागो, और जानकार श्रेष्ठ पुरुषों के सान्निध्य में ज्ञान प्राप्त करो। विद्वान्मनीषी जनों का कहना है कि ज्ञान प्राप्ति का मार्ग उसी प्रकार दुर्गम है जिस प्रकार छुरे के पैना किये गये धार पर चलना।

Prof MK Singh MBBS, MS

Professor and Ex-Head, Department of Ophthalmology
Chief, Regional Institute of Ophthalmology
Institute of Medical Sciences
Banaras Hindu University, Varanasi

Foreword

Foreword

प्रिय डॉक्टर सत्येंद्र जी
नमस्कार

अत्यंत हर्ष की बात है कि आप लोगों ने *COVID-19: Challenges Ahead* नामक पुस्तक को संपादित किया है। मुझे पूरा विश्वास है कि यह पुस्तक सभी लोगों के लिए बहुत ही उपयोगी रहेगी।

वैश्विक महामारी ने हमें अपनी पुरानी संस्कृति और सभ्यता की याद दिला दी है। भारतीय संस्कृति में प्रकृति कि पूजा की गई है। प्रकृति ही जीवन देती है और प्रकृति से मानव जाति को खिलवाड़ नहीं करना चाहिए।

कोरोना महामारी की वजह से लोग हाथ नहीं मिला रहे, गले नहीं मिल रहे, साफ सफाई का ध्यान रख रहे हैं और नमस्ते (प्रणाम) को अपना रहे हैं। प्रत्येक धर्म के लोगों का अपने अपने ईश्वर के प्रति आस्था बढ़ी है। कहने का तात्पर्य यह है कि प्रत्येक धर्म के लोगों ने इस बीमारी से छुटकारा पाने के लिए ईश्वर से प्रार्थना शुरू कर दी है। ऐसा लगता है इस बीमारी ने लोगो को भारतीय संस्कृति और सभ्यता की याद दिला दी है। अब लोग संस्कारित होने लगे हैं। यही भारतीय संस्कृति थी जिसको हमने पाश्चात्य सभ्यता की चकाचौंध में खो दिया था।

इस कथन के मध्य मुझे श्री रामचरितमानस की एक चौपाई याद आती हैं जिसमें गरुड़ जी कागभुसुंडि जी से प्रश्न पूछते हैं–

एक ब्याधि बस नर मरहिं ए असाधि बहु ब्याधि।

पीड़हिं संतत जीव कहुँ सो किमि लहै समाधि।।

अर्थात–एक ही रोग के वश होकर मनुष्य मर जाते हैं, फिर ये तो बहुत से असाध्य रोग हैं। ये जीव को निरंतर कष्ट देते रहते हैं, ऐसी दशा में वह समाधि (शांति) को कैसे प्राप्त करे?

अखिल विश्व यह मोर उपाया, सब पर मोही बराबर दाया।

सनातन संस्कृति में सभी को ईश्वर का बताया गया है और सभी पर उनकी बराबर कृपा बनी रहती है। हमें केवल जीवन के मूल्यों का पालन नैसर्गिक तरीके से करना है। मेरी ढ़ेरों शुभकामनाऐं आप सबके साथ है।

विजयेंद्र MBBS, MS, MCh (Paed Surgery)
Professor and Head
Department of Paediatric surgery
Indira Gandhi Institute of Medical Sciences, Patna
National President, National Medicos Organisation (NMO)

Foreword

COVID-19 is an infectious disease caused by newly discovered coronavirus. Majority of people infected with COVID-19 experience mild to moderate respiratory illness and recover without any special treatment. Elderly persons with co-morbid conditions are more likely to develop serious illness. At present time, there are no specific vaccines or treatment for COVID-19. However, there are many ongoing clinical trials evaluating potential treatments. All over the world health professionals and scientists have come together to accelerate the research to develop new norms and standards to contain the spread of coronavirus pandemic and to provide help to those who are affected. In our institute also, faculty members have come together and tried to share their knowledge and experience. They presented their efforts in form of this book. I sincerely hope that medical fraternity will find this book useful.

Prof RK Jain
Dean and Director
Institute of Medical Sciences
Banaras Hindu University
Varanasi

Foreword

In late December 2019, Wuhan city, China witnessed the outbreak of an unknown disease with an unidentified cause. Various cases were reported in hospitals about unexplainable pneumonia along with a past history of exposure to large seafood market of Wuhan city. Few days later, the causative agent was identified as ß-Coronavirus. The new virus was temporarily named the 2019-novel coronavirus (2019-nCoV) by the World Health Organization (WHO). Later, the pathogen was renamed severe acute respiratory syndrome coronavirus-2 (SARS-CoV-2) by International Committee on Taxonomy of Viruses and the disease was formally named coronavirus disease-2019 (COVID-19) by WHO.

The virus is responsible for the major cause of mortality across the world, in the past few months. The clinical features varies from asymptomatic to symptoms such as dry cough, fever, sore throat, difficulty in breathing, headache to severe acute respiratory syndrome. The severity of COVID-19 is not only caused by the viral infection but also due to the dysfunctional immune response of the host. This book *COVID-19: Challenges Ahead* provides an insight into the epidemiology, investigative modalities and clinical presentation of COVID-19 patients in India. The book elaborates on the paediatric, geriatric and critical care management of these patients. Surgical procedure in these patients needs different surgical practice and precautions are well covered. The emerging psychosocial issue associated with this pandemic requires attention and needs to be addressed by the medical fraternity. The challenges ahead by the practicing physicians and surgeons are well addressed using realistic facts, figures and evidence-based endeavours by two well-renowned surgeons Dr Satyendra K Tiwary and Dr Vishwambhar Singh.

This book will be very useful for surgeons, physicians, general practitioners and medical students. I congratulate both the editors and recommend this book to all medical fraternity.

Prof Puneet MS, DNB (Surg), MNAMS, FACS
Professor and Head
Department of Surgery
Institute of Medical Sciences
Banaras Hindu University
Varanasi, India

Preface

In the present times, when the whole world is facing a horrific pandemic of COVID-19, we here in Institute of Medical Sciences, Banaras Hindu University, Varanasi, were thinking that it may not reach us after its origin from Wuhan in China. Initial news from those area did not make us feel that the situation here may also reach the stage of lockdown. Then the news from Europe started coming and India too started gearing up for the same. And our preparation also started in smooth and big way to face the pandemic caused by novel coronavirus, probably a virus of origin from bats(?).

Since time immemorial, mankind has faced such circumstances multiple times in the history of evolution. But it has always come out with the solution. The human life on earth is blessed to have all the facilities for living a life. The environment in which we are born is good for living beings but we human beings do not take care of the environment and always try to manipulate one thing or other for our profit. But the correction factor of the Universe mostly plays a strong role and a limiting factor for such happening however appears. The dreaded COVID-19 which reached India on 30th of January made us all pondering how to combat with it. The initial reports were not very clear, and even not so now.

Lockdown of India begin on 22nd of March for physical distancing which was the only instrument available against the spread of virus at that time. The world was already engulfed in COVID-19 and presently almost all of the countries of world are struggling for an answer of this pandemic.

The information coming from the various levels need to be properly disseminated in the healthcare workers and the society. We are with less number of cases and deaths than the Western world. Either we have a better immunity or we have followed the lockdown very well. Some say that the strain of virus in India is also weak and different from the many parts of the world. But whatever the scenario, there are ever-changing guidelines appearing across the globe, so we thought to disseminate this knowledge properly to the healthcare workers by disseminating the guidelines presently available by various associations and government agencies. Some of the experiences may be shared by a few of the authors after work on the patients which were managed here or what we followed here to control the spread, identify and treat.

Presently the whole world is afraid of COVID-19, but mankind has always come with the solution for the same. We here in IMS BHU are doing whatever the guidelines have been given by the government of India and the other agencies, we are following the duty protocol as well as we are trying to come out with the book. As it is the need of the hour to tell what should be done. We, the authors, are devoted group of faculty members who played various roles during this phase.

There are various levels of hospitals in India and many medical students and doctors are working across India and will continue to work till the end of this pandemic but the basic knowledge must be acquainted by them. To overcome this, we started writing this book with a group of authors. This book will be a help to the mankind during this COVID-19. It will be of use for the future generations about how we faced this COVID-19, how the guidelines kept on changing, how the scenario kept on changing and how the doctors of that time, the scientist of that time, health workers of that time fought with COVID-19.

We are not having any previous knowledge about COVID-19, but some knowledge with the previous epidemics is helping us a lot, and this epidemic will be a lesson to the mankind, doctors, scientists and healthcare workers across the globe for coming years in future.

History repeats itself and every chapter has its significant for the future.

This book is also a tribute to all human life sacrificed during the pandemic. The corona warriors who lost their lives in serving mankind need to be respected by further developments to combat and overcome this pandemic.

With hope and light for the mankind.

ॐ।

भारत माता की जय।

Satyendra K Tiwary
Vishwambhar Singh

Contents

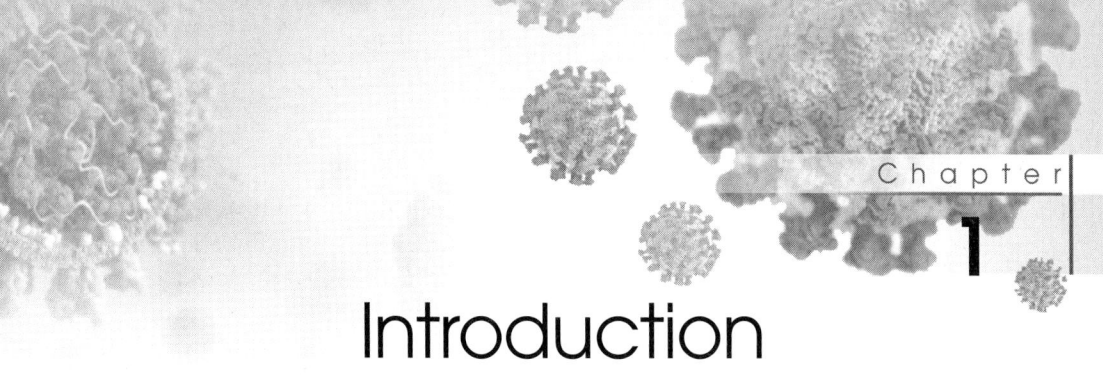

Introduction

Satyendra K Tiwary, Vishwambhar Singh

With the arrival of New Year 2020, alarming bell in health sector was ringing. On the last day of the year 2019, Coronavirus disease 2019 (COVID-19) was reported to WHO in the form of severe acute respiratory illness outbreak in Wuhan city, Hubei province, China.[1,2] It was notified as global health emergency just after 4 weeks on 30 January 2020 and within six weeks, it was officially a global pandemic on March 11 with declaration from WHO.[3]

SARS-CoV-2 nomenclature given on 11 February 2020 by International Committee on Taxonomy of Viruses, has changed the every aspect of life, health, work, planning and development globally with onset of its effect in the disease termed **COVID-19** (coronavirus disease 2019).[4] The name was chosen to avoid stigmatizing the virus' origins in terms of populations, geography, or animal associations.[5]

Considering the wings of COVID-19 engulfing the globe and a large population affected, aftermaths will be for decades just like scars imprinted by smallpox for the human beings. Whole exercise from a focal point or global perspective targets containment, control and cure of the disease. We are having only containment and control and no cure established till date which is a bitter truth to remember for caution as well as care in COVID-19.

A guideline has been issued by CDC with a recommendation that the general public gathering should not be more than 10 at a place at a time and face coverings with mask should be a routine when working in public places even by asymptomatic individuals to reduce the risk of transmission of COVID-19.[6] The CDC advises that non-pharmaceutical interventions (NPIs) will serve as the most important response strategy in attempting to delay viral spread and to reduce disease impact.[7]

Only preventive tools are with us in COVID-19 crisis and care, so every aspect of containment and breakdown of chain of transmission is probably most definitive target in this pandemic.

The CDC has also provided recommendations for individuals who are at high risk of COVID-19-related complications, including older adults and persons who have serious underlying health conditions (e.g. heart disease, diabetes, lung disease).[8]

CLINICAL FEATURES

There is always myriad possibility of presentations in COVID-19, which may be either asymptomatic or with mild symptoms in most cases but severe manifestations needing ventilator support with higher possibility of death are also within the spectrum of the disease during an usual incubation period of 2 days to 2 weeks in most cases.[9,10]

Cough and shortness of breath or difficulty in breathing plus at least two of the following symptoms may indicate COVID-19:[11]

- Fever
- Chills
- Repeated shaking with chills
- Muscle pain
- Headache
- Sore throat
- New loss of taste or smell

Other reported symptoms have included the following:

- Fatigue
- Sputum production
- Diarrhoea
- Malaise
- Respiratory distress

The most common serious manifestation appears to be pneumonia due to acute lung injury.

DIAGNOSIS

COVID-19 is considered a possibility in:

1. Patients with respiratory tract symptoms and newly onset fever, or
2. In patients with severe lower respiratory tract symptoms with no clear cause.

Suspicion is increased, if such patients have been in an area with community transmission of SARS-CoV-2 or have been in close contact with an individual with confirmed or suspected COVID-19 in the preceding 14 days.

Microbiologic testing is required for definitive diagnosis. Patients who do not require emergency care are encouraged to contact their healthcare provider over the phone. Patients with suspected COVID-19 who present to a healthcare facility should prompt infection-control measures. They should be evaluated in a private room with the door closed (an airborne infection isolation room is ideal) and asked to wear a surgical mask. All other standard contact and airborne precautions should be observed, and treating healthcare personnel should wear eye protection.[12]

MANAGEMENT

The antiviral drug Remdesivir gained emergency use authorization (EUA) from the FDA on May 1, 2020, based on preliminary data showing a faster time to recovery of hospitalized patients with severe disease.[13] Numerous other antiviral agents, immunotherapies, and vaccines continue to be investigated and developed as potential therapies.

In addition, infected patients should receive supportive care to help alleviate symptoms. Vital organ function should be supported in severe cases.[14]

No vaccine is currently available for SARS-CoV-2. Avoidance is the principal method of deterrence.

Numerous collaborative efforts to discover and evaluate effectiveness of antivirals, immunotherapies, monoclonal antibodies, and vaccines have rapidly emerged. Guidelines and reviews of pharmacotherapy for COVID-19 have been published.[15,16]

Numerous clinical guidelines have been issued for COVID-19 as summarized below:

- *COVID-19 Enforcement Policy for Sterilizers, Disinfectant Devices, and Air Purifiers (FDA, 2020):* 2020 COVID-19 guidance for industry and FDA staff.

- *OSHA Guidance on Preparing the Workplace for COVID-19 (2020):* 2020 guidance on preparing the workplace for coronavirus disease 2019 (COVID-19) by the Occupational Safety and Health Administration (OSHA).

- *COVID-19 Breast Cancer Patient Triage Guidelines (CPBCC):* Guidelines on surgical triage of patients with breast cancer by the COVID-19 Pandemic Breast Cancer Consortium.

- *Procedures in Known/Suspected COVID-19 (ASA, 2020):* 2020 guidelines on performing procedures on patients with known or suspected COVID-19 by the American Society of Anesthesiologists (ASA).

- *COVID-19-Related Airway Management Clinical Practice Guidelines (SIAARTI/EAMS, 2020):* 2020 clinical practice guidelines from the SIAARTI Airway Research Group and the European Airway Management Society on coronavirus disease 2019 (COVID-19)-related airway management.

- *Surviving Sepsis Campaign: Guidelines on the Management of Critically Ill Adults with Coronavirus Disease 2019 (COVID-19):* Panel consisting of 36 experts from 12 countries compiled 54 evidence-based statements for clinicians caring for patients with severe COVID-19 infection.

- *Belgium Task Force on supportive care and antiviral/immunologic treatment of hospitalized patients with suspected or confirmed COVID-19 (2020):* 2020 interim clinical guidance by the Belgium Task Force for supportive care and antiviral/immunologic therapy for adults with suspected or confirmed coronavirus disease 2019 (COVID-19).

- *COVID-19 Ventilation Clinical Practice Guidelines (2020):* COVID-19 ventilation clinical practice guidelines by the European Society of Intensive Care Medicine and the Society of Critical Care Medicine.

- *Guidance on Obstetric COVID-19 (ISUOG, 2020):* Guidance on the management of COVID-19 infection during pregnancy, childbirth, and the neonatal period, from the International Society of Ultrasound in Obstetrics and Gynecology.

- *Control of COVID-19 in Nursing Homes Guidelines (2020):* 2020 guidelines on infection control and prevention of COVID-19 in nursing homes by the Centers for Medicare and Medicaid Services (CMS).

- *FDA Face Mask and Respirator Policy in COVID-19 (2020):* 2020 guidelines on enforcement policy for face masks and respirators by the US Food and Drug Administration (FDA).
- *Rapid COVID-19 Clinical Practice Guidelines (2020):* Rapid COVID-19 clinical practice guidelines by Wuhan University Novel Coronavirus Management and Research Team and China International Exchange and Promotive Association for Medical and Health Care.
- *Guidance on Cardiac Implications of COVID-19 (ACC, 2020):* 2020 guidance by the American College of Cardiology regarding the cardiac implications of COVID-19.
- *COVID-19 Guidance for Ophthalmologists (AAO, 2020):* 2020 COVID-19 guidance for urgent and nonurgent patient care in ophthalmology.
- *Guidance on Containing Spread of COVID-19 (CMS, 2020):* Guidance for hospitals on how to identify at-risk patients, screen for COVID-19, and monitor or restrict health care facility staff, from the Centers for Medicare and Medicaid Services.
- *COVID-19 Sample Collection and Testing: Clinical Practice Guidelines (CDC, 2020):* 2020 clinical practice guidelines from the Centers for Disease Control and Prevention on the collection, handling, and testing of specimens for the diagnosis of coronavirus disease 2019 (COVID-19).
- *Guidelines for Evaluating and Testing Persons Under Investigation for COVID-19 (CDC, 2020):* 2020 clinical practice guidelines on evaluating and testing persons under investigation for coronavirus disease 2019 (COVID-19) by the Centers for Disease Control and Prevention (CDC).

These guidelines are being formulated on war footage evolving rapidly and this list will be swelling more and more as the time will pass in the hope of some good news on COVID-19 war front. But there are certain facts helping always to control the disease. If transmission is prevented or minimized that is probably the only definitive armamentarium available with us to fight the disease. We cannot give definitive treatment but only supportive treatment available for different organ systems and high mortality in high viraemia cases with acute lung injury.

The most common ways in which COVID-19 can spread are:

- Coughing and sneezing without covering your mouth as this can spread the droplets containing the virus in the air.
- Coming into contact with a person who is already carrying the virus.
- Coming into contact with any object which contains the virus and then touching your nose or mouth.

The primary mode of transmission is through respiratory droplets generated when an infected person coughs, sneezes, or talks. Droplets that settle on the eyes, nose, or mouth of a person in close proximity lead to the transmission of infection. Transmission can also occur by touching the face with contaminated hands. Respiratory droplets do not remain suspended in the air for long; hence, a distance of six feet away from an infected person may be considered safe.

First and foremost golden rule in survival during war with COVID-19 is to maintain a distance of 6 feet to avoid direct droplet exposure as safe distance of six feet may be barrier to control the disease. Almost 80% of droplets generated fall within 1.5 feet but a distance of 6 feet reduces risk as 99.9% droplets are contained in this range.

Second golden rule in survival against COVID-19 is sanitization of hands with washing and hygiene maintenance. Contact with contaminated surfaces (fomites) and subsequent transfer to the face by touch may also be an important mode of transmission which is broken down with this second tool. Contaminated metal, glass, or plastic surfaces that may remain infective for several days should not be touched at all, but frequent handwashing and hygiene maintenance with sanitizer helps a lot and cuts this mode of transmission by contaminated surfaces.

Third golden rule is safety mask application to minimize risk. It can be of great advantage in breaking the chain of transmission as one may not get protected completely from getting infection but biggest gain is wearing mask limits the capacity to transmit the infected droplets to the others, due to barrier role of the mask. Airborne transmission, distinct from droplet infection, is characterized by viruses that drift through the air. It is still not clear, if airborne transmission occurs or not but considering the other respiratory infections transmitted by air, this mode cannot be ruled out completely. This should be taken care by safety masks application including surgical masks and N-95 masks.

These three golden rules of safe distance with separation by 6 feet, sanitization of hands by hygiene maintenance with frequent washing and safety mask over face covering nose and mouth prevent the danger and reduce the risk of getting infected or transmitting to others.

Fourth golden rule is screening which will save others from being hit by the virus. If there are any alarming clinical manifestations in the form of cough, fever, dyspnoea, loss of taste or smell, sore throat, headache, body ache, immediate attention with screening to detect earliest infection, quarantine, isolate and prevent further infection transmission in the society. Thermal scanners are effective in mass screening to detect raised body temperature with detection and work-up in suspicious cases. So, golden rule of screening will prevent further transmission from the source, if detected in time the infected cases.

Fifth golden rule is safety culture development for long-term benefit to the society and mankind not only to fight COVID-19 but any similar large-scale pandemic hitting in future. Cultural changes are most difficult, take time but set the value and long-term benefits are more to stand high at the time of crisis. Parts of cultural values and changes are like wearing masks, making masks at the local level, care of self and others, handwashing habits, physical distancing, and earlier identification of the ill and subsequent treatment, care, and support. Exercises, physical activity, healthy dietary habits and self-restrain are parts of culture which pay in long term in output. These are long-term goals to be set as part of cultural shift in the society.

In summary, *five golden rules* **for every warrior in war against COVID-19:**

1. Safe distance with six feet separation.
2. Sanitization of hands, washing and hygiene maintenance.
3. Safety mask covering face including nose and mouth.
4. Screening suspects with symptoms, signs and use of scanner.
5. Set cultural development for values and safety.

This five-point follow-up for survival in COVID-19 era sets the gear and momentum to do definite work at different levels with exploration of all aspects of the disease in terms of every aspect in the developmental and clinical history of the disease.

▌REFERENCES

1. Gallegos A. WHO declares public health emergency for novel coronavirus. Medscape Medical News. Available at https://www.medscape.com/viewarticle/924596. January 30, 2020; Accessed: May 2, 2020.

2. CDC. 2019 Novel Coronavirus, Wuhan, China. CDC. Available at https://www.cdc.gov/coronavirus/2019-ncov/about/index.html. January 26, 2020; Accessed: May 2, 2020.

3. Ramzy A, McNeil DG. WHO Declares Global Emergency as Wuhan Coronavirus Spreads. The New York Times. Available at https://nyti.ms/2RER70M. January 30, 2020; Accessed: May 2, 2020.

4. Gorbalenya AE. Severe acute respiratory syndrome-related coronavirus – The species and its viruses, a statement of the Coronavirus Study Group. Available at https://doi.org/10.1101/2020.02.07.937862. February 11, 2020; Accessed: May 2, 2020.

5. WHO Director-General's remarks at the media briefing on 2019-nCoV on 11 February 2020. Available at https://www.who.int/dg/speeches/detail/who-director-general-s-remarks-at-the-media-briefing-on-2019-ncov-on-11-february-2020. February 11, 2020; Accessed: May 2, 13, 2020.

6. CDC. Coronavirus Disease 2019 (COVID-19): Recommendations for Cloth Face Covers. Centers for Disease Control and Prevention. Available at https://www.cdc.gov/coronavirus/2019-ncov/prevent-getting-sick/cloth-face-cover.html. April 3, 2020; Accessed: May 2, 2020.

7. Ferguson NM, Laydon D, Nedjati-Gilani G, Imai N, Ainslie K, Baguelin M, et al. Impact of non-pharmaceutical interventions (NPIs) to reduce COVID-19 mortality and healthcare demand. Imperial College COVID-19 Response Team. Available at https://www.imperial.ac.uk/media/imperial-college/medicine/sph/ide/gida-fellowships/Imperial-College-COVID19-NPI-modelling-16-03-2020.pdf. 2020 Mar 16; Accessed: May 2, 2020.

8. Centers for Disease Control and Prevention. Coronavirus Disease 2019 (COVID-19): People at Higher Risk. Centers for Disease Control and Prevention. Available at https://www.cdc.gov/coronavirus/2019-ncov/specific-groups/high-risk-complications.html. March 8, 2020; Accessed: May 2, 2020.

9. CDC. 2019 Novel Coronavirus, Wuhan, China: Symptoms. CDC. Available at https://www.cdc.gov/coronavirus/2019-ncov/about/symptoms.html. January 26, 2020; Accessed: May 2, 2020

10. Lauer SA, Grantz KH, Bi Q, Jones FK, Zheng Q, Meredith HR, et al. The Incubation Period of Coronavirus Disease 2019 (COVID-19) From Publicly Reported Confirmed Cases: Estimation and Application. *Ann Intern Med*. 2020 Mar 10. [Medline].

11. CDC. Symptoms of Coronavirus. CDC. Available at https://www.cdc.gov/coronavirus/2019-ncov/symptoms-testing/symptoms.html. March 20, 2020; Accessed: April 28, 2020.

12. CDC. 2019 Novel Coronavirus, Wuhan, China: Interim Healthcare Infection Prevention and Control Recommendations for Patients Under Investigation for 2019 Novel Coronavirus. CDC. Available at https://www.cdc.gov/coronavirus/2019-ncov/infection-control.html. January 18, 2020; Accessed: January 27, 2020.

13. FDA. Coronavirus (COVID-19) Update: FDA Issues Emergency Use Authorization for Potential COVID-19 Treatment. fda.gov. Available at https://www.fda.gov/news-events/press-announcements/coronavirus-covid-19-update-fda-issues-emergency-use-authorization-potential-covid-19-treatment. May 01, 2020; Accessed: May 01, 2020

14. CDC. 2019 Novel Coronavirus, Wuhan, China: Prevention & Treatment. CDC. Available at https://www.cdc.gov/coronavirus/2019-ncov/about/prevention-treatment.html. January 26, 2020; Accessed: January 27, 2020

15. Sanders JM, Monogue ML, Jodlowski TZ, Cutrell JB. Pharmacologic Treatments for Coronavirus Disease 2019 (COVID-19): A Review. *JAMA*. 2020 Apr 13.

16. Barlow A, Landolf KM, Barlow B, Yeung SYA, Heavner JJ, Claassen CW, et al. Review of Emerging Pharmacotherapy for the Treatment of Coronavirus Disease 2019. *Pharmacotherapy*. 2020 Apr 7.

Basic Infection Prevention and Control Practices

Tuhina Banerjee, Rahul Garg

COVID-19 is an emerging infectious disease of global public health concern. Efforts to control the COVID-19 epidemic are likely to require an evidence-based, multifactorial approach. Infection prevention and control (IPC) practices are of critical importance in protecting the functioning of healthcare services and mitigating the impact on vulnerable populations. In the face of the rapidly spreading disease and a large number of infected people, there is an urgent need for proactively perform infection control measures among healthcare workers (HCWs).

PRINCIPLES OF IPC STRATEGIES ASSOCIATED WITH HEALTHCARE FOR SUSPECTED COVID-19

To achieve the highest level of effectiveness in the response to the COVID-19 outbreak using the infection control practices, a dedicated and trained team supported by local administrative authorities is most crucial. The team represents the core committee members which includes an infection control officer (clinical microbiologist or infectious disease physician), infection control nurses, infection control laboratory technicians, and data entry operators, who actually performs the various functions at ground level and effectively implement the infection control programme in the hospital.

IPC strategies to prevent the transmission of COVID-19 in healthcare settings include the following:[1]

1. Ensuring triage, screening, and source control (isolating patients with suspected COVID-19).
2. Applying standard infection control precautions for all patients and implementing transmission-based precautions (droplet and contact and, whenever applicable, airborne precautions).
3. Implementing administrative controls.
4. Using environmental and engineering controls.

Standard infection control precautions and transmission-based precautions must be used when managing patients with suspected or confirmed COVID-19.

Standard Infection Control Precautions

It includes the basic infection prevention and control measures necessary to reduce the risk of transmission of infectious agents from the sources. Sources include blood and other body fluids, secretions and excretions (excluding sweat), non-intact skin or mucous membranes, and any equipment or items in the care environment. It should be used by all the HCWs for all the patients, all the time.

Transmission-Based Precautions

They are applied when standard infection control precautions alone are insufficient to prevent cross-transmission of an infectious agent. They are additional infection control precautions required when caring for a patient with a known or suspected infectious agent.

Transmission-based precautions are categorized by the route of transmission of the infectious agent.

Routes of Transmission of COVID-19

Current information suggests that the two main routes of transmission of the COVID-19 virus are respiratory droplets and contact.[2] Respiratory droplets are generated when an infected person coughs or sneezes. Any person who is in close contact (within 1 m) with someone who has respiratory symptoms (coughing, sneezing) is at risk of being exposed to potentially infective respiratory droplets. Droplets may also on surfaces where the virus could remain viable; thus, the immediate environment of an infected individual can serve as a source of transmission (contact transmission).

Ensuring Triage, Screening, and Source Control

Triage includes a system for assessing all patients at admission, allowing for early screening of possible COVID-19 and immediate isolation of patients with suspected disease in an area separate from other patients (source control). To facilitate the early identification of such cases, healthcare facilities should:[1]

a. Encourage HCWs to have a high level of clinical suspicion.

b. Establish a well-equipped triage station at the entrance to the facility, supported by trained staff.

c. Institute the use of screening questionnaires according to the updated case definition.

d. Post signs in public areas reminding symptomatic patients to alert HCWs.

APPLYING STANDARD INFECTION CONTROL PRECAUTIONS FOR ALL PATIENTS

Standard precautions include hand and respiratory hygiene, the use of appropriate personal protective equipment (PPE) according to a risk assessment, injection safety practices, safe biomedical waste management, proper linens, environmental cleaning, and sterilization of patient-care equipment.[3]

Hand Hygiene Practices[4]

Hand hygiene is the single most effective and critical element of standard infection control precautions in both the healthcare settings and the community. The ability of hand hygiene, including handwashing or the use of alcohol-based hand rubs (ABHR) to prevent infections is related to reductions in the number of viable pathogens that transiently contaminate the hands. Centers for Disease Control and Prevention (CDC) recommends the use of ABHR with greater than 60% ethanol or 70% isopropanol as the preferred form of hand hygiene in healthcare settings. Hand hygiene must be performed immediately before every episode of direct patient care and after any activity or contact that potentially results in hands becoming contaminated, including the removal of personal protective equipment (PPE), equipment decontamination, and waste handling.

ABHR must be available for all staff as near to point of care as possible, where this is not practical, personal dispensers should be used. The technique for use of ABHR to decontaminate hands must be carried out thoroughly and for a period sufficient to inactivate the virus, i.e. 20 to 30 seconds.

The indications for using ABHRs are:

a. During routine clinical rounds and handling the patient.

b. If the hands are not visibly dirty.

c. If hands are not contaminated with blood or body fluids.

While the technique for handwashing with soap and water must be carried out thoroughly and for a period sufficient to inactivate the virus, i.e. 40 to 60 seconds.

The few indications for using handwash in the healthcare facility are:

a. Hands are visibly dirty or feel dirty or sweaty, contaminated with blood, or body fluids.

b. After using the washroom or toilets.

c. Before handling medication or food.

The steps of hand hygiene procedure (Figs 2.1 and 2.2) were formulated by WHO based on the observations of various studies which showed that there are areas of the hands which are frequently missed, if all steps not followed properly.

Respiratory and Cough Hygiene—'Catch It, Bin It, Kill It'

Patients, HCWs, and visitors should be encouraged to minimize the spread of COVID-19 through good respiratory hygiene measures:[1]

- Disposable, single-use tissues, if available, should be used to cover the nose and mouth when sneezing, coughing, or wiping and blowing the nose. Used tissues should be disposed of promptly in the nearest waste bin.
- Always cover every cough, sneeze and nasal blowing with your shoulder or inner side of the elbow.
- If hands are used, it should be cleaned (using soap and water, if possible, otherwise using ABHR) after coughing, sneezing, using tissues, or after any contact with respiratory secretions and contaminated objects.

HOW TO HAND RUB

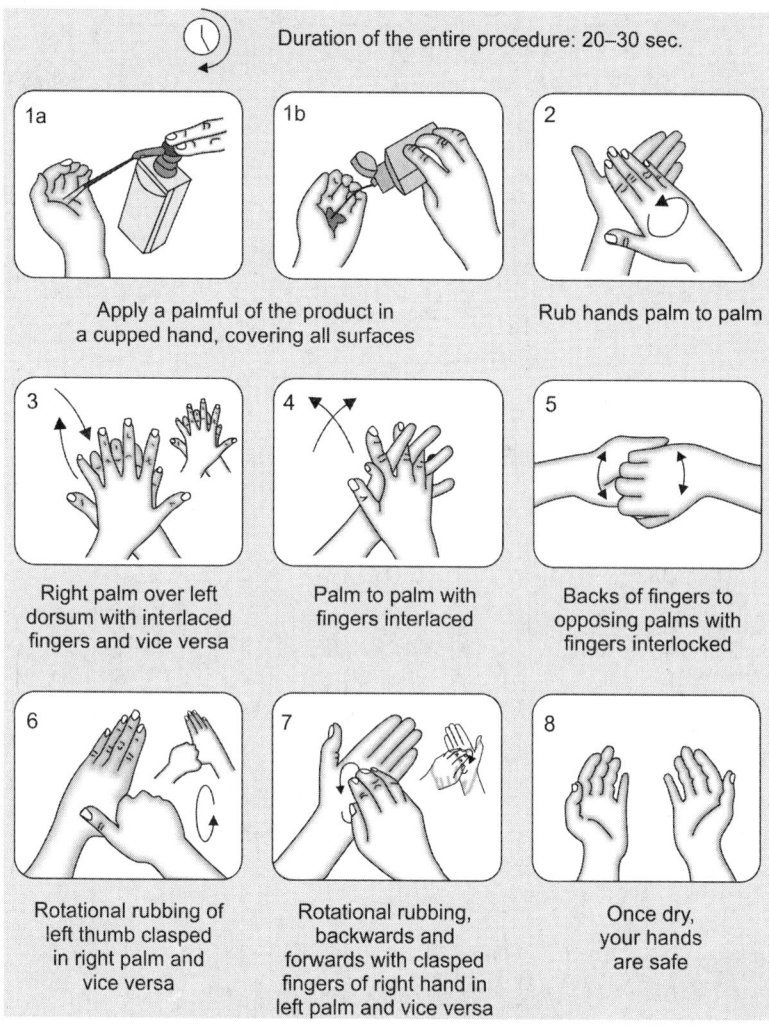

Duration of the entire procedure: 20–30 sec.

1a	**1b**	**2**
Apply a palmful of the product in a cupped hand, covering all surfaces		Rub hands palm to palm
3	**4**	**5**
Right palm over left dorsum with interlaced fingers and vice versa	Palm to palm with fingers interlaced	Backs of fingers to opposing palms with fingers interlocked
6	**7**	**8**
Rotational rubbing of left thumb clasped in right palm and vice versa	Rotational rubbing, backwards and forwards with clasped fingers of right hand in left palm and vice versa	Once dry, your hands are safe

Fig. 2.1: Hand rub steps (*Source:* WHO)

- Encourage patients and HCWs to keep hands away from the eyes, mouth, and nose.
- In common waiting areas or during transportation, symptomatic patients should be provided a surgical face mask, to minimize the dispersal of respiratory secretions and reduce environmental contamination.
- Practice no-touch greetings in the hospital like namaste or hello.
- Never touch lift buttons with your fingers. Always use your elbows to press elevator buttons.
- Maintain 1 meter (2 arms) social distance (Fig. 2.3):
  - If you have cough/sneeze (Fig. 2.4)
  - From people with respiratory symptoms
  - From contacts of corona cases who are on quarantine

HOW TO HANDWASH (Duration 40–60 sec)

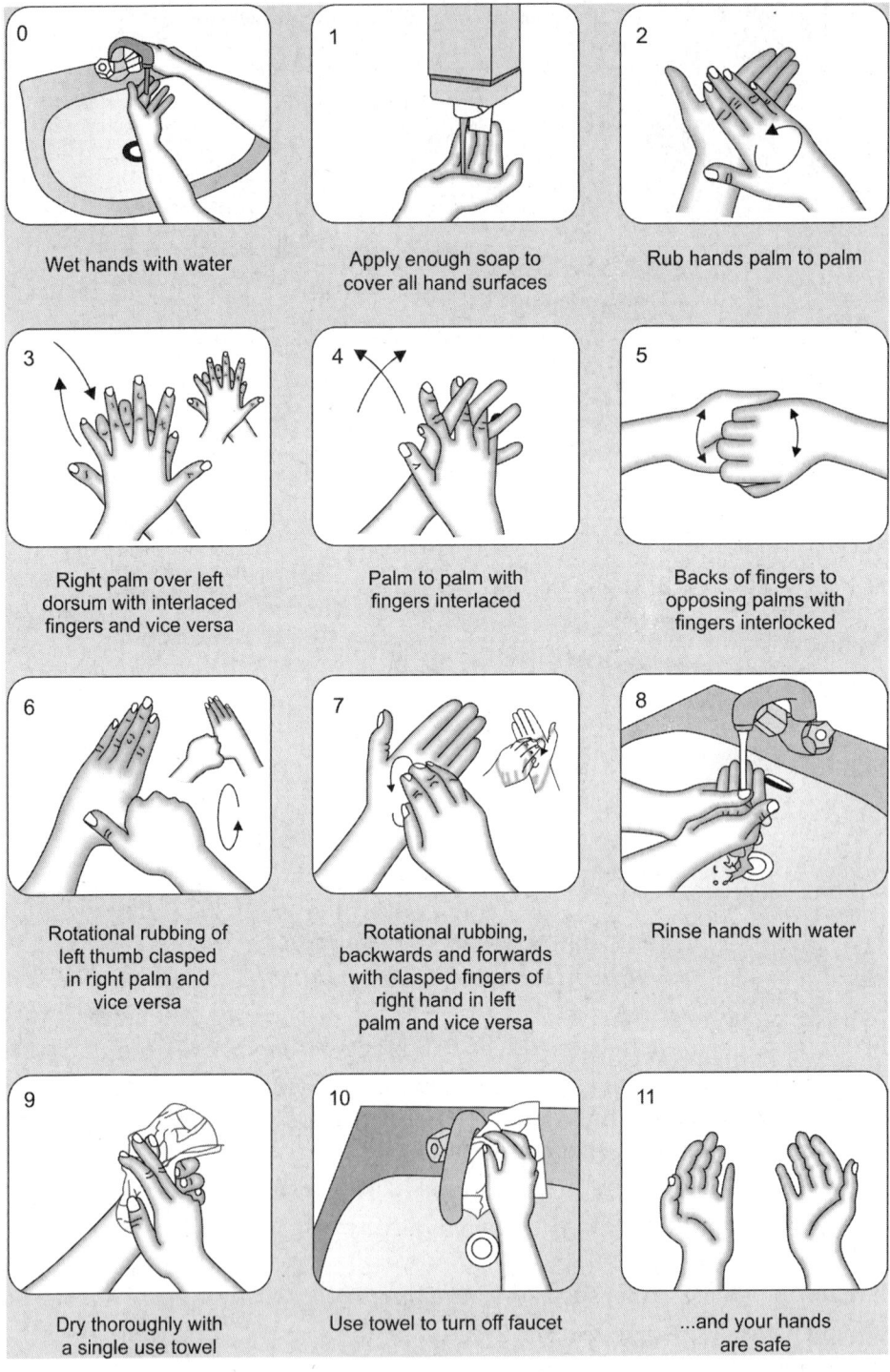

0 Wet hands with water	**1** Apply enough soap to cover all hand surfaces	**2** Rub hands palm to palm
3 Right palm over left dorsum with interlaced fingers and vice versa	**4** Palm to palm with fingers interlaced	**5** Backs of fingers to opposing palms with fingers interlocked
6 Rotational rubbing of left thumb clasped in right palm and vice versa	**7** Rotational rubbing, backwards and forwards with clasped fingers of right hand in left palm and vice versa	**8** Rinse hands with water
9 Dry thoroughly with a single use towel	**10** Use towel to turn off faucet	**11** ...and your hands are safe

Fig. 2.2: Handwash steps (*Source:* World Health Organization)

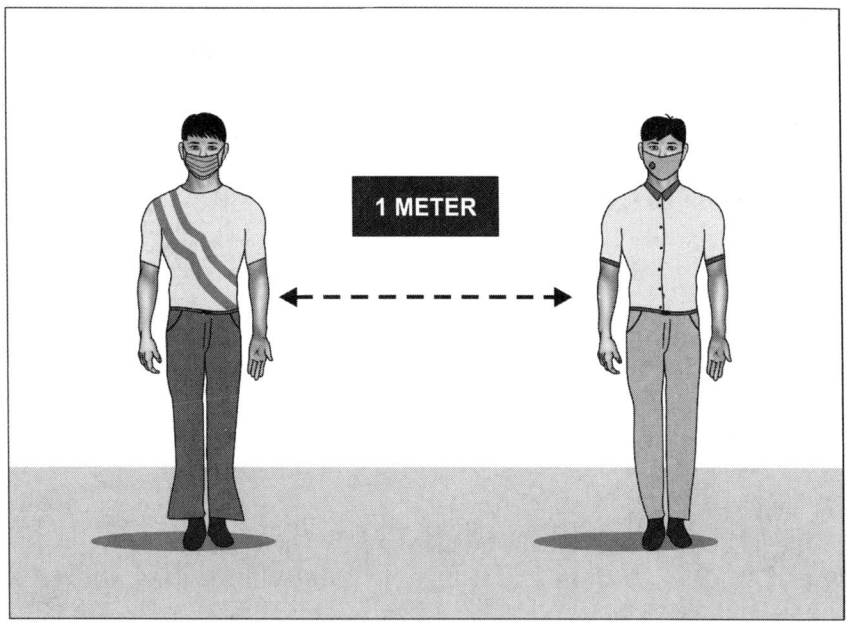

Fig. 2.3: Social distancing (*Source:* Centers for Disease Control and Prevention)

STOP THE SPREAD OF CORONAVIRUS

Nose blowing, sneezing and coughing etiquette

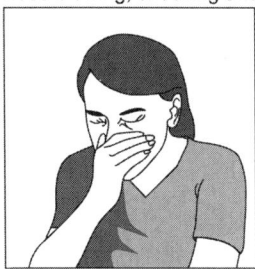 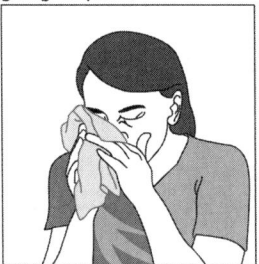 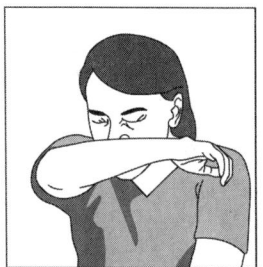

Do not cough or sneeze in your hands ✗ | Use a tissue and dispose immediately ✓✓ | If do not have tissue: Cough or sneeze into your upper sleeve ✓

After coughing, sneezing or blowing your nose

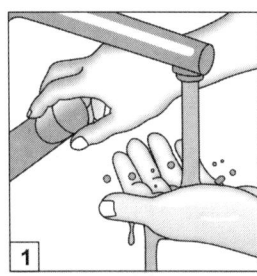 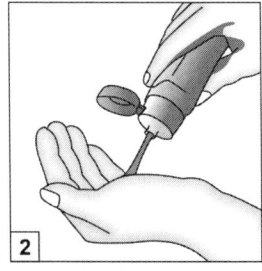 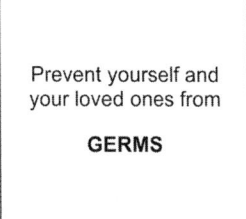

1

2

Wash your hands with soap and water | Disinfect visually clean hands with alcohol-based handrub | Prevent yourself and your loved ones from **GERMS**

Fig. 2.4: Respiratory etiquette (*Source:* Centers for Disease Control and Prevention)

Personal Protective Equipment for COVID-19[5]

Personal protections include two aspects: Wearing protective equipment and applying universal precautions. Personal protective equipment (PPE) are protective gear designed to safeguard the health workers by minimizing the exposure to a biological agent. Components of PPE are goggles for eye protection, face mask, gloves, coverall/gowns (with or without aprons), headcover, and shoe cover.

Although the use of PPE is the most visible control used to prevent the spread of infection, it is only one of the IPC measures and should not be relied on as a primary prevention strategy. In the absence of effective administrative and engineering controls, PPE has limited benefits. Given the global PPE shortage, strategies that can facilitate optimal availability like minimizing the need for PPE in healthcare settings, ensuring rational and appropriate use of PPE should be utilized.

Minimize the Need for PPE

1. Restrict visitors to the corona ward.
2. Restrict HCWs from entering the corona ward, if they are not involved in direct care. Streamline the workflow and reduce steps that require face-to-face interaction with the patient.
3. Screening area: Restrict HCWs evaluating suspected cases of COVID-19 disease, one HCW can screen, others can maintain distance and interact; thus, minimizing the need for these individuals to go to healthcare facilities for evaluation.
4. Use physical barriers to reduce exposure to the COVID-19 virus. This approach can be implemented in areas of the healthcare setting where patients will first present, such as triage area, the registration desk at the emergency department, or at the pharmacy window where medication is collected.
5. Postpone elective, non-urgent operations, and hospitalizations, reduce the frequency of visits for chronic patients, apply telemedicine solutions where possible.
6. Cohort confirmed COVID-19 patients without coinfection with other transmissible microorganisms in the same room to streamline the workflow and facilitate extended use of PPE.

Ensure PPE Use is Rationalized and Appropriate

PPE should be used based on the risk of exposure; will vary according to the setting and type of personnel and activity (Table 2.1). The overuse/misuse of PPE will have a further impact on supply shortages.

1. Direct contact without aerosol-generating procedures of corona patients (suspected/confirmed) should use the following PPE: Gowns, gloves, surgical mask, and eye protection (goggles or face shield).
2. Aerosol-generating procedures (e.g. tracheal intubation, open suctioning, non-invasive positive pressure ventilation (BiPAP and CPAP), tracheostomy, cardiopulmonary resuscitation, manual ventilation before intubation, bronchoscopy, airway suction, chest physiotherapy, nebulizer treatment, sputum induction, collection of specimens); HCWs should use gowns, gloves, eye protection (goggles or face shield), respirators (N95) and apron.

3. General public, without respiratory symptoms, need no medical mask. Wearing mask creates a false sense of security that can lead to the neglect of other essential preventive measures such as hand hygiene, social distancing.
4. General public with respiratory symptoms should wear a medical mask and seek medical care.

Table 2.1: Recommended PPE during the outbreak of COVID-19, according to the setting, personnel, and type of activity

No.	Settings	Activity	Type of PPE or procedure	Remarks
1.	HCWs in screening/ triage area	Preliminary screening not involving direct contact (history taking, interacting, temperature recording)	• Maintain physical distance of at least 1 m • Use medical mask • Gloves	Provide medical mask to suspected COVID-19 patient Perform hand hygiene and have the patient perform hand hygiene
2.	Patient room/ ward	HCWs providing direct care to COVID-19 patients, in the absence of aerosol generating procedures	• Medical mask • Gown • Gloves • Eye protection (goggles or face shield) • Perform hand hygiene	
		HCWs providing direct care to COVID-19 patients in settings where **aerosol-generating procedures** are frequently in place	• Respirator N95 or FFP2 or FFP3 standard, or equivalent • Gown • Gloves • Eye protection • Apron • Perform hand hygiene	
		Cleaners entering the room of COVID-19 patients	• Medical mask • Gown • Heavy-duty gloves • Eye protection (if the risk of splash from organic material or chemicals is anticipated) • Closed work shoes • Perform hand hygiene	
3.	Areas of transit where patients are not allowed	All staff, including healthcare workers	• Maintain physical distance of at least 1 m	

Contd.

Table 2.1: Recommended PPE during the outbreak of COVID-19, according to the setting, personnel, and type of activity (Contd.)

No.	Settings	Activity	Type of PPE or procedure	Remarks
	including administrative areas		• No PPE required • Perform hand hygiene	
4.	Ambulance driver	Involved only in driving the patient with suspected COVID-19 disease and the driver's compartment is separated from the COVID-19 patient	• Maintain physical distance of at least 1 m • Medical mask • Perform hand hygiene	Provide medical mask to suspected patient
		Assisting with loading or unloading patient with suspected COVID-19	• Medical mask • Gowns • Gloves • Goggles • Perform hand hygiene	Provide medical mask to suspected patient
5.	Laundry	Linen transport	• Medical mask • Gloves	
		Linen cleaning (after pre-soaking in 0.5% hypochlorite)	• Medical mask • Gloves	
6.	Home	Patients with symptoms suggestive of COVID-19	• Maintain physical distance of at least 1 m • Provide medical mask • Hand and respiratory hygiene	
		Caregiver providing direct care or when handling stool, urine, or waste from COVID-19 patient being cared for at home	• Gloves • Medical mask • Apron (if risk of splash is anticipated) • Perform hand hygiene	Provide medical mask to the patient

Face Masks and Respirators[6]

Respiratory protection reduces the inhalation of aerosols and, therefore, is essential when there is risk of droplet transmission. There are two types of PPE available for respiratory protection: Face masks and respirators.

Face masks: Face masks include *surgical masks*, which are fluid resistant, and *procedure masks*, which are not fluid resistant.

In the three-layered surgical masks, the innermost layer is made up of an absorbent material that absorbs moisture from the wearer's breath, the middle layer is made up of a melt-blown material that acts as a filter, and the outer layer is made up of material that repels liquid. The pleats are intended to increase the surface area so that the nose and the chin can also be adequately covered. It is held in place by strings either looping around the ears or tied behind.

Surgical masks are intended to be used only once and then safely disposed of. They should never be washed and reused. The life of a surgical mask varies according to its use, but generally lasts for between 4 and 6 hours depending on the environmental humidity, temperature and volume of air breathed. It is important to know how to wear a surgical mask and how to remove it (Fig. 2.5).

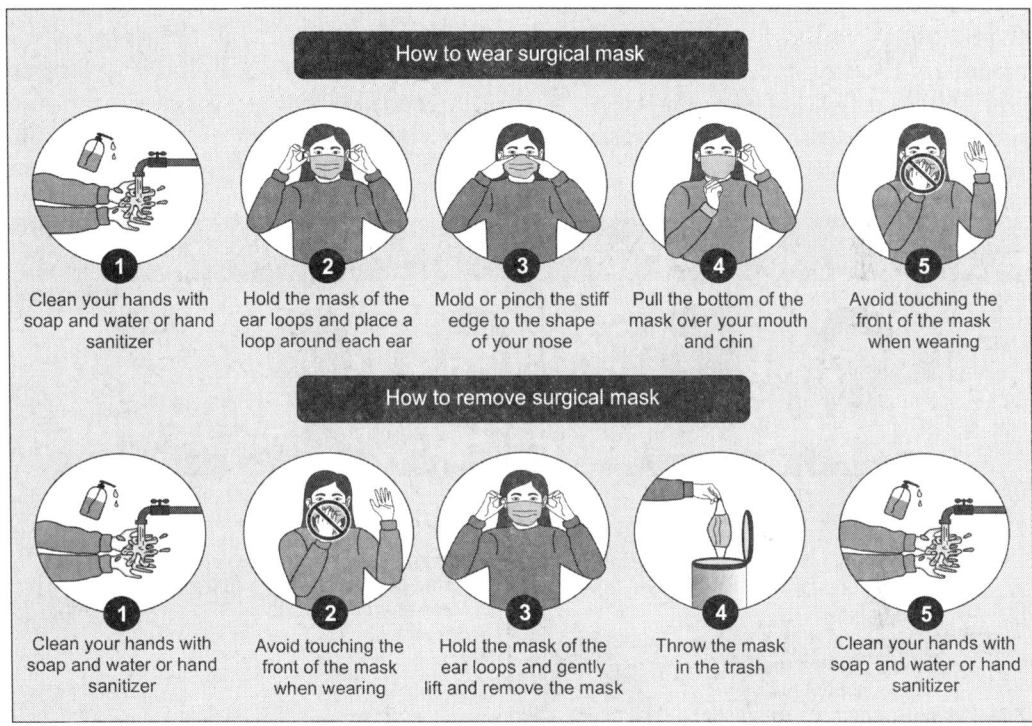

Fig. 2.5: How to wear and remove surgical mask (*Source:* Centers for Disease Control and Prevention)

Medical masks should be reserved for HCWs. The use of masks in the community may create a false sense of security, with neglect of other essential measures, such as hand hygiene practices and physical distancing, and may lead to touching the face under the masks and under the eyes, resulting in the risk of infection.[7]

Respirator mask (N95, FFP2, FFP3): A respirator mask is a tight-fitting mask with a filtration system that prevents the wearer from being exposed to noxious particles, gases, oils, or microorganisms, including bacteria, viruses, and fungi. It has two specific characteristics, viz:

1. An air-filtering system that prevents the passage of noxious substances and microorganisms from entering inside the respiratory tract, and

2. A tight fit, so that air does not leak from the sides into the nose and mouth.

The filter of the N95 mask is made up of millions of microfibres of polypropylene layered on top of each other that have been permanently electrostatically charged.

The electrical charge is necessary to retain its ability to filter microorganisms or microparticles.

Respiratory masks are certified into N, R, or P depending on their ability to offer resistance to oil-based particles by the National Institute of Occupational Safety and Health (NIOSH). N stands for 'not oil-resistant', these masks can only be used for particles that do not contain oil. R stands for 'somewhat resistant to oil', and P stands for 'strongly oil-proof'. N is further divided into N95, N99, N100 depending on the filtration efficacy. N95 means that this mask can filter off at least 95% of particles which are >0.3 microns, while N99 means it can filter off 99% of these particles. While the European Union classifies respirator masks into FFP1, FFP2, and FFP3 where FFP stands for filtering face piece. N95 is roughly equivalent to FFP2 and N99 is roughly equivalent to FFP3 masks. The HCW must follow the correct technique of donning (Fig. 2.6) and doffing the N95 respirator; otherwise, it may not provide adequate respiratory protection.

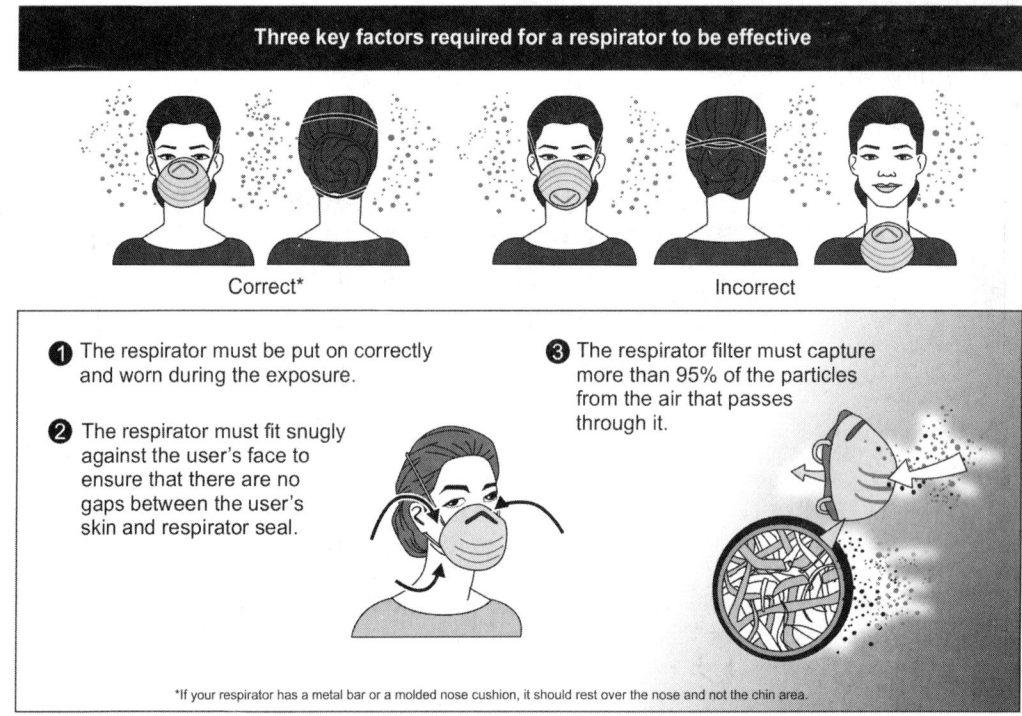

Fig. 2.6: Effective way to wear N95 respirator (*Source:* Centers for Disease Control and Prevention)

Fit check for N95 respirators: HCWs must perform fit checking every time they put on an N95 respirator to ensure if it is properly fitted and functional.
1. Placement: The respirator is placed on the face and tied over the head and at the base of the neck.
2. Sealing: N95 mask is compressed to ensure a seal across the face, cheeks, and bridge of the nose.
3. The positive pressure seal of the N95 mask is checked by gently exhaling. If air escapes, the N95 mask needs to be adjusted.

4. The negative pressure seal of the N95 mask is checked by gently inhaling. If the N95 mask is not drawn in towards the face or air leaks around the face seal; the N95 mask is readjusted and the process is repeated.

5. If still not proper, then its respirator should be checked for any defect or damage.

Mask Management (Fig. 2.7)

For any type of mask, appropriate use and disposal are essential to ensure that they are effective and to avoid any increase in transmission. The following information on the correct use of masks are derived from practices in healthcare settings.

- Place the mask carefully, ensuring it covers the mouth and nose, and tie it securely to minimize any gaps between the face and the mask.
- Avoid touching the mask while wearing it. Do not allow tangling of mask around the neck.
- Remove the mask using the appropriate technique: Do not touch the front of the mask but untie it from behind.
- After removal or whenever a used mask is inadvertently touched, clean hands using an ABHR or soap and water, if hands are visibly dirty.
- Replace masks as soon as they become damp with a new clean, dry mask. Discard the mask in yellow bin.

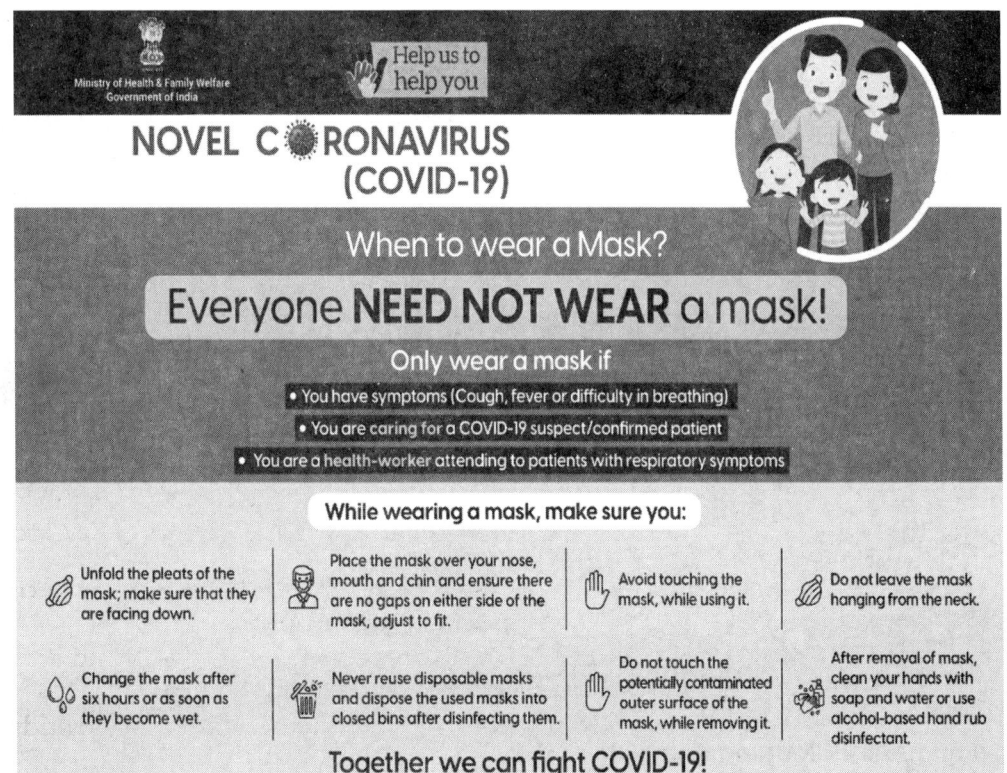

Fig. 2.7: Mask management (*Source:* MoHFW, New Delhi)

Donning and Doffing of PPE[8]

The purpose of PPE use can be fulfilled only when they are worn in the correct sequence (donning) and removed in the correct sequence (doffing) and proper steps are followed for each of the PPE while donning and doffing (Fig. 2.8).

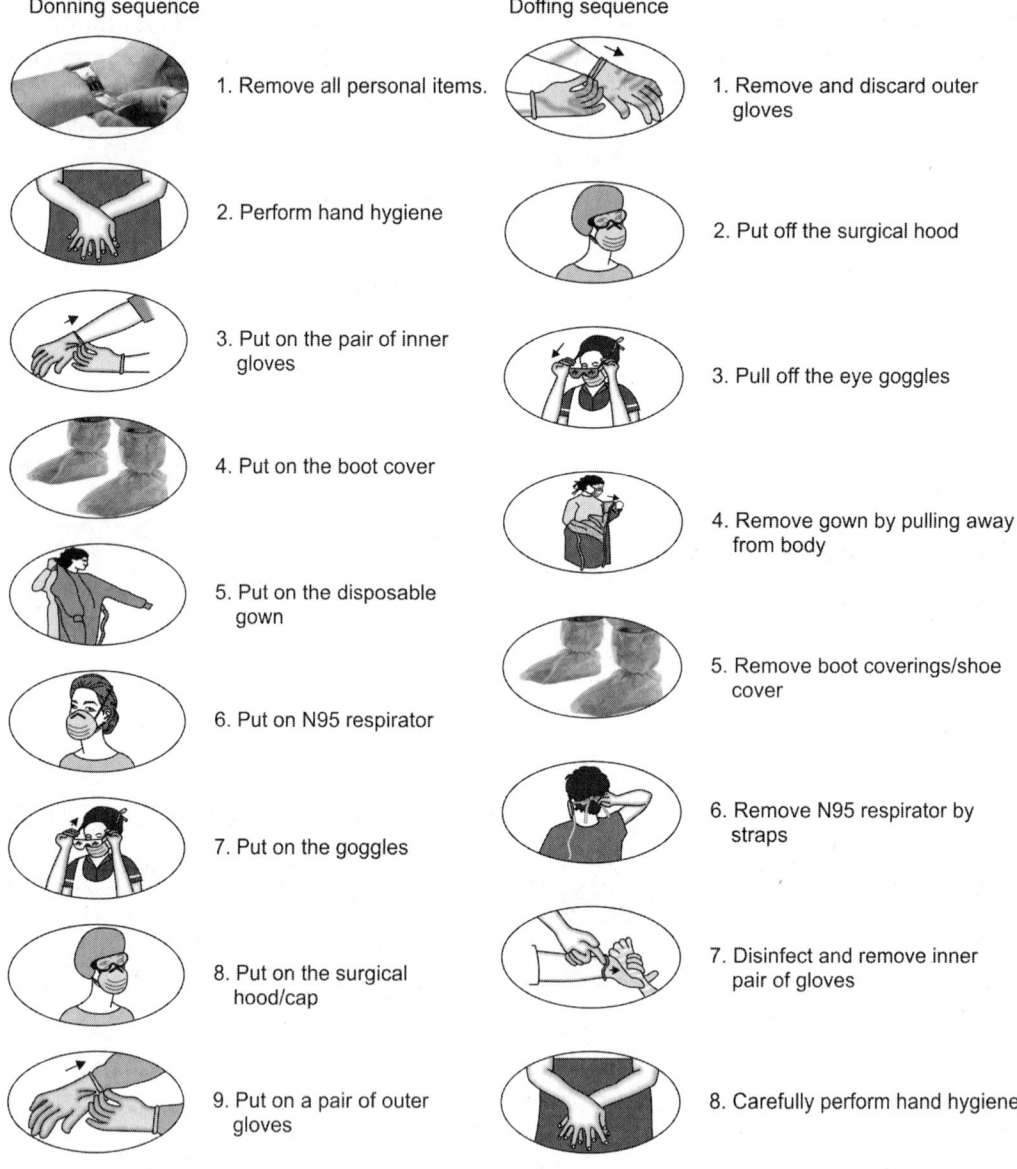

Donning sequence

1. Remove all personal items.

2. Perform hand hygiene

3. Put on the pair of inner gloves

4. Put on the boot cover

5. Put on the disposable gown

6. Put on N95 respirator

7. Put on the goggles

8. Put on the surgical hood/cap

9. Put on a pair of outer gloves

Doffing sequence

1. Remove and discard outer gloves

2. Put off the surgical hood

3. Pull off the eye goggles

4. Remove gown by pulling away from body

5. Remove boot coverings/shoe cover

6. Remove N95 respirator by straps

7. Disinfect and remove inner pair of gloves

8. Carefully perform hand hygiene

Fig. 2.8: Sequence of donning and doffing

Environmental Cleaning and Disinfection[1,9]

SARS-CoV-2 can potentially survive in the environment for several hours/days.[10] Therefore, transmission can occur by direct contact with infected people and indirect contact with surfaces in the immediate environment or with objects used on the infected person. Thus, it is important to follow proper hand hygiene and clean and disinfect environmental surfaces consistently and correctly, thus minimizing the risk of spread of infection.

Many disinfectants are active against enveloped viruses, such as the SARS-CoV-2, including commonly used hospital disinfectants. Currently, the WHO recommends using (Fig. 2.9):

- 70% ethyl alcohol to disinfect high-touch surfaces having frequent hand contacts, such as door handles, mobile phones, bed rails, IV stand, etc.
- Freshly prepared sodium hypochlorite at 1% (equivalent to 10000 ppm) with a contact time of 10 min for disinfecting low-touch surfaces having minimal hand contacts such as the floor, ceilings, and walls.

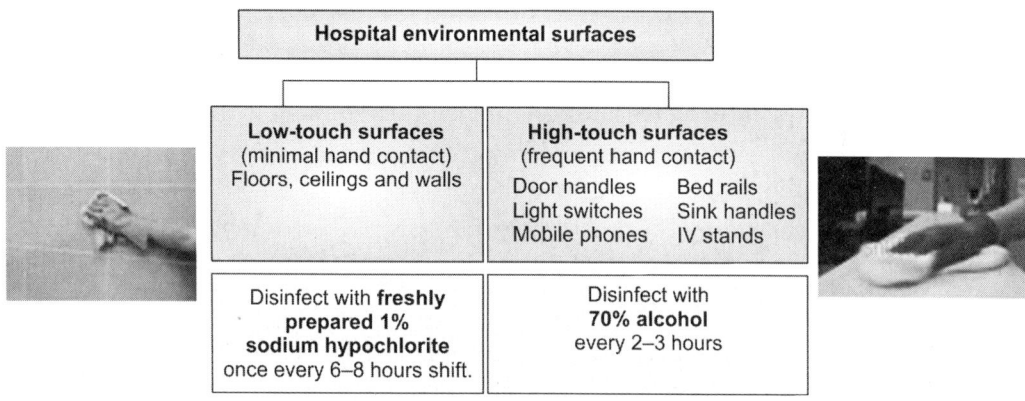

Fig. 2.9: Environmental cleaning and disinfection of low-touch and high-touch surfaces

General Advisory for Cleaning and Disinfection (Table 2.2)

1. Designated housekeeping staff should be well trained in cleaning environmental surfaces, hand hygiene, and PPE.
2. Never use a broom in any hospital area. Always do wet mopping with detergent and disinfectant (hypochlorite).
3. The housekeeping staff must wear appropriate PPE (heavy-duty gloves, surgical mask, goggles/face shield, gown, and boots or closed shoes) before starting cleaning or disinfection.
4. Use fresh cleaning cloths at the start of each cleaning session.
5. Change cleaning clothes between each patient zone (i.e. use a new cleaning cloth for each patient bed). For example, in a multi-bed intensive care unit, the fresh cloth is required for every bed/incubator.
6. Remove gross soil (visible to naked eye) before cleaning and disinfection.
7. Thoroughly wet (soak) a fresh cleaning cloth in the environmental cleaning solution.
8. Never shake mop heads and cleaning clothes—it disperses dust or droplets that could contain microorganisms.
9. Use a three-bucket system (for disinfection): One bucket contains the detergent or cleaning solution; one contains rinse water and one the disinfectant or disinfectant solution.

10. Clean and disinfect all surfaces. This includes horizontal, vertical, and contact patients and surrounding surfaces.

11. Cleaning sequence: Always clean from top-to-down sequence, i.e. ceiling-based equipment first, walls, then floor-based equipment, and lastly the floor.

12. When cleaning the floor, begin at the end farthest from the door and move towards the door (in to out).

13. The cleaning staff should always move from clean to unclean areas and never vice versa.

14. When cleaning individual equipment: Clean from top to down.

15. Proceed in a methodical, systematic manner to avoid missing areas.

16. Only leave the room when cleaning is completed.

17. Remove PPE and perform hand hygiene before leaving the patient environment and discard in the appropriate biomedical waste bin.

18. Never leave soiled mop heads and cleaning clothes soaking in buckets.

19. Do not use disinfectants spray-on potentially highly contaminated areas as it may create splashes that can further spread the virus.

20. Maintain a daily cleaning checklist under the supervision of the nursing staff.

Table 2.2: Cleaning area and disinfectant

COVID isolation room/ quarantine room, triage area	Disinfectant	Contact time	Frequency
High-touch surfaces	70% alcohol	—	Every 2–3 hrly
Floor	Clean (detergent and water) and then hypochlorite 1%	10 min	Every 6–8 hrly
Wall, ceiling	Hypochlorite 1%	10 min	Once daily
Toilet	Clean (detergent and water) and then hypochlorite 1%	10 min	Every 6–8 hrly

Soiled Linen Laundry for COVID-19[1]

1. Never carry soiled linen against the body.

2. Hand hygiene and PPE (surgical mask, heavy-duty gloves, plastic apron, and boots).

3. A dedicated laundry area should be there for cleaning soiled bedding, towels, and clothes from patients with COVID-19.

4. Soiled linen should be placed in clearly labelled, leak-proof bags or containers, carefully removing any solid excrement and putting in a covered bucket to dispose off in the toilet.

5. If the washing machine is there:
   - Wash at 60–90°C with laundry detergent followed by soaking in 0.5% sodium hypochlorite for approximately 30 minutes and dried.

6. If no machine washing is there:
   - Soaked in hot water with soap/detergent in a large drum.

  – Use a stick to stir and avoid splashing.
  – Empty the drum and soak linen in 0.5% sodium hypochlorite for approximately 30 minutes.
7. Rinse with clean water and let linen dry fully in the sunlight.

Biomedical Waste Management for COVID-19[11]

COVID-19 corona isolation wards need to follow these steps to ensure safe handling and disposal of biomedical waste generated during patient care and in the clinical laboratories. Segregation and disposal of biomedical waste (BMW) should be followed as BMWM rules, 2016 as amended (Table 2.3).

Table 2.3: Different colour coding for hospital items and disposal methods of BMW

Colour-coded bag/box	Items	Disposal method
Yellow	Infectious non-plastic, non-sharp	Incineration
Red	Infectious plastic, non-sharp	Autoclave or microwave
White sharp box	Sharp (metal)	Sharp pit
Blue box	Glass, metal implants	Autoclave

However, the following additional steps need to be kept in mind.
- Keep **separate dedicated colour-coded bins/bags/containers** in corona wards/ICU and should be labelled **'COVID-19 waste'.**
- Use **double-layered bags** (using two bags) should be used for the collection of waste from COVID-19 wards/ICU to ensure adequate strength and no-leaks.
- Inside the COVID isolation room/ICU, all waste should be considered as infectious waste; and therefore, no waste should be discarded in the black bag.
- Transport to a final treatment facility: Keep 'COVID-19 waste' separately in a temporary storage room before handing over to an authorized staff of treatment facility.
- Disinfection: The inner and outer surface of bags/containers/collection bins/trolleys should be disinfected with 1% sodium hypochlorite.
- General waste not having contamination should be disposed off as solid waste (black bag).
- Maintain a separate record of waste generated from COVID-19 wards/ICU.
- PPEs: Depute dedicated housekeeping staff and use adequate PPEs: Three-layered mask, apron/gowns, gloves, and gumboots.
- Dedicated vehicle: Treatment facility should use a dedicated vehicle for transport of COVID-19 waste; however, separate label as **'COVID-19 waste'** is not necessary and the vehicle should be disinfected with 1% hypochlorite after every trip to the healthcare facility.
- The PPE should be disposed off as:
  – Gloves, plastic apron, goggles—red
  – Non-plastic items such as mask, gown, cap, shoe cover—yellow bag

Dead Body Management for COVID-19[12]

The main route of transmission of COVID-19 is through droplets. Therefore, it is unlikely to have an increased risk of COVID infection from a dead body to health workers or family members who follow standard precautions while handling the body. Only the lungs of dead COVID patients, if handled during an autopsy, can be infectious. However, till now there is no such acceptable scientific data that COVID-19 cannot spread through dead bodies, except the lungs. The dead bodies are considered to be a source of infection in several infectious diseases.

All staff identified to handle dead bodies in the isolation area, mortuary, ambulance and those workers in the crematorium/burial ground should be trained in the infection prevention control practices.

Overall recommendations by Ministry of Health and Family Welfare (MoHFW) are:

1. Body bag: One body bag, robust leak-proof of 150 μm thickness is needed.
2. Viewing of the body is allowed with standard precautions.
3. Embalming of the dead body should not be allowed.
4. Hygienic preparation—either not allowed, or allowed with appropriate PPEs.
5. Autopsy—need to be avoided as much as possible.
6. Final treatment—either cremation or cuffing depending upon the religious practice.

Standard precautions to be followed by HCWs while handling dead bodies of COVID-19 are:

1. Perform hand hygiene.
2. Use of personal protective equipment (e.g. gown, gloves, masks, eyewear, headcover, and shoe cover).
3. Safe handling of sharps.
4. Disinfect bag housing dead body; instruments and devices used on the patient.
5. Disinfect linen with 1% sodium hypochlorite. Clean and disinfect environmental surfaces.

IMPLEMENTING ADMINISTRATIVE CONTROLS[1,13]

The administrative measures related to HCWs are:

1. Provision of adequate IPC training for HCWs.
2. Ensuring an adequate patient-to-staff ratio.
3. Establishing a surveillance process for acute respiratory infections potentially caused by COVID-19 virus among HCWs.
4. Ensuring that HCWs and the public understand the importance of promptly seeking medical care.
5. Monitoring HCW compliance with standard precautions and providing mechanisms for improvement as needed.
6. Ensuring adequate supplies of PPE and hand rubs.
7. Preventing overcrowding, especially in emergency departments.

USING ENVIRONMENTAL AND ENGINEERING CONTROLS[1]

These controls address the basic infrastructure of the healthcare facility and aim to ensure adequate ventilation in all areas in the healthcare facility, as well as adequate environmental cleaning. Additionally, separation of at least 1 metre should be maintained between all patients. Both spatial separation and adequate ventilation can help reduce the spread of many pathogens in the healthcare setting.

REFERENCES

1. World Health Organization. Infection prevention and control during health care when novel coronavirus (nCoV) infection is suspected: Interim guidance, 19 March 2020.
2. World Health Organization. Advice on the use of masks in the context of COVID-19: Interim guidance, 6 April 2020. World Health Organization; 2020.
3. Siegel JD, Rhinehart E, Jackson M, Chiarello L, Health Care Infection Control Practices Advisory Committee. 2007 guideline for isolation precautions: Preventing transmission of infectious agents in health care settings. American Journal of Infection Control 2007 Dec;35(10):S65.
4. Boyce JM, Pittet D. Guideline for hand hygiene in health-care settings: Recommendations of the Healthcare Infection Control Practices Advisory Committee and the HICPAC/SHEA/APIC/IDSA Hand Hygiene Task Force. Infection Control and Hospital Epidemiology. 2002 Dec;23(S12): S3–40.
5. World Health Organization. Rational use of personal protective equipment for coronavirus disease (COVID-19) and considerations during severe shortages: Interim guidance, 6 April 2020. World Health Organization; 2020.
6. World Health Organization. Advice on the use of masks in the context of COVID-19: Interim guidance, 6 April 2020. World Health Organization; 2020.
7. Feng S, Shen C, Xia N, Song W, Fan M, Cowling BJ. Rational use of face masks in the COVID-19 pandemic. The Lancet Respiratory Medicine 2020 Mar 20.
8. Centers for Disease Control and Prevention. Interim infection prevention and control recommendations for patients with suspected or confirmed coronavirus disease 2019 (COVID-19) in healthcare settings. COVID-19. 2020 Mar 19.
9. CDC and ICAN. Best Practices for Environmental Cleaning in Healthcare Facilities in Resource-Limited Settings. Atlanta, GA: US Department of Health and Human Services, CDC; Cape Town, South Africa: Infection Control Africa Network; 2019. Available at: https://www.cdc.gov/hai/prevent/resource-limited/environmental-cleaning.html and http://www.icanetwork.co.za/icanguideline2019/.
10. van Doremalen N, Bushmaker T, Morris DH, Holbrook MG, Gamble A, Williamson BN, Tamin A, Harcourt JL, Thornburg NJ, Gerber SI, Lloyd-Smith JO. Aerosol and surface stability of SARS-CoV-2 as compared with SARS-CoV-1. New England Journal of Medicine 2020 Mar 17.
11. Guidelines for Handling, Treatment and Disposal of Waste Generated during Treatment/Diagnosis/ Quarantine of COVID-19 Patients – Revision 2 dated 18/04/2020.
12. World Health Organization. Water, sanitation, hygiene, and waste management for the COVID-19 virus: Interim guidance, 23 April 2020. World Health Organization; 2020.
13. Guidance O. COVID-19: Guidance for infection prevention and control in healthcare settings. Version 1.0. Department of Health and Social Care (DHSC). Public Health Wales (PHW), Public Health Agency (PHA) Northern Ireland, Health Protection Scotland (HPS) and Public Health England. 2020.

Epidemiology of COVID-19

Sunil Kumar, Sachchidanand

BURDEN OF DISEASE

Worldwide more than 9.3 million confirmed cases of COVID-19 have been reported. In India, first case of 2019–20 coronavirus pandemic was reported on 30 January 2020. As of 23rd June 2020, The Ministry of Health and Family Welfare have confirmed a total of 4,56,115 cases, 2,58,684 recoveries and 14,476 deaths in the country.[1] Going by current trend and according to experts, the cases are likely to peak in July. In India, the infection rate of COVID-19 is reported to be 1.7, significantly lower than in the worst affected countries.[2]

AGENT FACTOR

Agent: Coronavirus is a single-stranded RNA virus belonging to the family of Coronaviridae and subfamily Orthocoronavirinae. Some of viruses causing illness in humans and others circulate among animals, including camels, cats, bats, etc. The aetiologic agent responsible for present outbreak of COVID-19 is SARS-CoV-2 which is a novel coronavirus. Many experts feel that COVID-19 is a laboratory-made virus. Different experts have different opinions regarding its country of origin.[3]

Mode of transmission: COVID-19 can be transmitted directly through droplet when susceptible host is within 1 metre (3 feet) distance. Indirectly it can be transmitted through fomites. Unclean hands and fingers also transmit the infection only by mechanical transmission.[1] In an analysis of 75,465 COVID-19 cases in China, airborne transmission was not reported.[4]

Source of infection: A case (either subclinical or clinical) of coronavirus is the source of infection. Fomites are another important source.[4] Studies have shown that the COVID-19 virus can survive for up to 72 hours on plastic and stainless steel, less than 4 hours on copper and less than 24 hours on cardboard.[5] This may vary under different conditions (e.g. type of surface, temperature or humidity of the environment).

Predisposing factors: Lowered immunity, comorbidities, overcrowding and extremes of ages are predisposing factors for COVID.[1]

Carrier state: Subclinical and incubatory carries have been found in COVID-19.

Portal of entry: The virus commonly enters through nose, mouth and eyes.[1] It can enter through any serous membrane.

Portal of exit: The virus is excreted by coughing and sneezing of an infected patient. It has been found in stool also.[1]

Period of communicability: Definite period of communicability is not known at this time. Some studies have suggested transmission as early as five days before onset of symptoms.[6]

Reservoir of infection: Coronaviruses are a large family of viruses that are common in animals. Occasionally, people get infected with these viruses which may then spread to other people. For example, SARS-CoV was associated with civet cats and MERS-CoV is transmitted by dromedary camels.[7] Possible animal sources of COVID-19 have been found in zoo animals and pets. There has been one instance of a dog being infected in Hong Kong.

Incubation period: Current estimates of the incubation period of 2019-nCoV range from 2–14 days. In some rare cases, it has been observed to be up to 30 days. The mean incubation period was 5.1 days in case of COVID-19 pneumonia.[8]

Secondary attack rate: Assuming that all secondary infections were generated by a single primary case, which is probable given the short-term nature of the exposure events, would imply an SAR among close contacts of 35%.[6]

HOST FACTORS

Age: All ages coming in contact with the source of infection has been found to be affected. Observed mortality rate is high among extremes of ages. In first 425 cases with confirmed nCoV pneumonia at Wuhan, China; the median age was 59 years. The elderly patients (above 60 years old) present the highest risk to COVID-19, even greater than having any comorbidity. On the other hand, it seems that younger adult patients (30–39 years old) present some protection.[9]

Gender: Males have shown higher rates of infection. But it may be due to high mobility rate of males.

Race: All races have been found to be infected.

Religion and caste: No religion or caste has shown the predilection for COVID-19 infection. High rate of infectivity observed in a religion may be attributed to overcrowding and immunity level.

Socioeconomic status: Infection rate and mortality rate have been high in developed country at initial stage of pandemic. It may be attributed to less effective control on social distancing measures, such as public transport, flight, etc.

Immunity: Level of immunity has definite inverse relationship with the COVID-19 infection and mortality. Comorbidity lowers the immunity. Cardiovascular disease appears to be the riskiest, which is higher than having a chronic respiratory disease.[10] Patients with previous cardiovascular metabolic diseases, cancer may face a greater risk of developing into the severe condition and the comorbidities can also greatly affect the prognosis of the COVID-19. On the other hand, COVID-19 can, in turn, aggravate the damage to the heart.[6]

Nutrition: Overnourished as well as undernourished have high chance of getting infection.

Personal hygiene: Personal hygiene, especially hand hygiene is one of the most important determining factors for getting COVID infection.

ENVIRONMENTAL FACTORS

Environmental factors like overcrowding, poor ventilation, close habitation will increase COVID-19 transmission.[11]

Seasonal fluctuations: Hot and humid climate seems to be protective against COVID-19.

Cyclic fluctuations and secular trend: This is a novel coronavirus. An outbreak of coronavirus had occurred in Guangdong province, China in 2002–03. But it was an SARS COVID-1.

FREQUENCY OF DISEASE

Mortality rates: The case fatality rate varies from country to country. In India, it is 3.3%. The case fatality rate is as low as 0.3% in Germany, while it as high as 9.4% in Netherland.[12]

Morbidity rates: The rate at which COVID-19 cases has been doubling in India is slower than several other countries such as the USA, Italy, Spain and the UK. Data from the health ministry and Worldometer, a website that records confirmed cases of infection and deaths globally, said that in India coronavirus cases doubled from 500 to 1,000 in five days and then took four days to reach 2,000. It took just three days for coronavirus cases in the country to double and reach the 4,000 mark but six days for the tally to reach 8,000. Then the doubling rate was eight days when the tally reached 16,000 and 10 days as it hit the 32,000 mark.[13]

TRANSMISSION OF COVID-19

Transmission of coronaviruses can occur via respiratory secretions. Nosocomial transmission has been documented in COVID-19. A brief overview of available evidence on transmission from symptomatic, presymptomatic and asymptomatic people infected with COVID-19 has been summarized below.

Symptomatic Transmission

As per definition, a symptomatic COVID-19 case is a case who has developed signs and symptoms compatible with COVID-19 virus infection. Symptomatic transmission refers to transmission from a person while they are experiencing symptoms. Data from published epidemiology and virologic studies provide evidence that COVID-19 is primarily transmitted from symptomatic people to others who are in close contact through respiratory droplets, by direct contact with infected persons, or by contact with contaminated objects and surfaces. Data from clinical and virologic studies that have collected repeated biological samples from confirmed patients provide evidence that shedding of the COVID-19 virus is highest in upper respiratory tract (nose and throat) early in the course of the disease. That is, within the first 3 days from onset of symptoms. Preliminary data suggests that people may be more contagious around the time of symptom onset as compared to later on in the disease.[14]

Presymptomatic Transmission

The incubation period for COVID-19, which is the time between exposure to the virus (becoming infected) and symptom onset, is on average 5–6 days, however, can be up to 14 days. During this period, also known as the 'presymptomatic' period, some infected persons can be contagious. Therefore, transmission from a presymptomatic case can occur before symptom onset. In a small number of case reports and studies, presymptomatic transmission has been documented through contact tracing efforts and enhanced investigation of clusters of confirmed cases. This is supported by data suggesting that some people can test positive for COVID-19 from 1–3 days before they develop symptoms. Thus, it is possible that people infected with COVID-19 could transmit the virus before significant symptoms develop. It is important to recognize that presymptomatic transmission still requires the virus to be spread via infectious droplets or through touching contaminated surfaces.[14]

Asymptomatic Transmission

An asymptomatic laboratory-confirmed case is a person infected with COVID-19 who does not develop symptoms. Asymptomatic transmission refers to transmission of the virus from a person, who does not develop symptoms. There are a few reports of laboratory-confirmed cases that are truly asymptomatic, and to date, there has been no documented asymptomatic transmission. This does not exclude the possibility that it may not occur. Asymptomatic cases have been reported as part of contact tracing efforts in some countries. WHO regularly monitors all emerging evidence about this critical topic and will provide an update as more information becomes available.[14]

CASE DEFINITIONS

Suspect Case

- A patient with acute respiratory illness, fever and at least one sign/symptom of respiratory disease (e.g. cough, shortness of breath), and a history of travel to or residence in a country/area or territory reporting local transmission of COVID-19 disease during the 14 days prior to symptom onset.
- A patient/healthcare worker with any acute respiratory illness and having been in contact with a confirmed COVID-19 case in the last 14 days prior to onset of symptoms.
- A patient with severe acute respiratory infection, fever and at least one sign/symptom of respiratory disease (e.g. cough, shortness of breath) and requiring hospitalization and with no other aetiology that fully explains the clinical presentation.
- A case for which testing for COVID-19 is inconclusive.[15]

Laboratory-Confirmed Case

A person with laboratory confirmation of COVID-19 infection, irrespective of clinical signs and symptoms.

CONTACT

A contact is a person that is involved in any of the following:

- Providing direct care without proper personal protective equipment (PPE) for COVID-19 patients.
- Staying in the same close environment of a COVID-19 patient (including workplace, classroom, household, gatherings).
- Travelling together in close proximity (1 m) with a symptomatic person who later tested positive for COVID-19.[15]

Types of Contact

High Risk

- Touched body fluids of the patient (respiratory tract secretions, blood, vomit, saliva, urine, faeces)
- Had direct physical contact with the body of the patient including physical examination without PPE.
- Touched or cleaned the linens, clothes, or dishes of the patient.
- Lives in the same household as the patient.
- Anyone in close proximity (within 3 feet) of the confirmed case without precautions.
- Passenger in close proximity (within 3 feet) of a conveyance with a symptomatic person who later tested positive for COVID-19 for more than 6 hours.[15]

Low Risk

- Shared the same space (same class for school/worked in same room/similar and not having a high-risk exposure to confirmed or suspect case of COVID-19).
- Travelled in same environment (bus/train/flight/any mode of transit) but not having a high-risk exposure.[15]

REFERENCES

1. *"Home | Ministry of Health and Family Welfare | GOI"*. *www.mohfw.gov.in. Retrieved 23 June, 2020.*
2. https://en.wikipedia.org/wiki/COVID-19_pandemic_in_India. *Retrieved 1 May, 2020*
3. Cascella M, Rajnik M, Cuomo A, Dulebohn SC, Di Napoli R. Features, evaluation and treatment coronavirus (COVID-19). In *Statpearls [internet]*. StatPearls Publishing, 2020.
4. China Ong SW, Tan YK, Chia PY, Lee TH, Ng OT, Wong MS, et al. Air, surface environmental, and personal protective equipment contamination by severe acute respiratory syndrome coronavirus 2 (SARS-CoV-2) from a symptomatic patient. JAMA 2020 Mar 4.
5. https://www.who.int/news-room/q-a-detail/q-a-coronaviruses. *Retrieved 1 May, 2020.*
6. https://www.publichealthontario.ca/-/media/documents/ncov/covid-wwksf/what-we-know-communicable-period-mar-27-2020.pdf?la=en. *Retrieved 1 May, 2020.*
7. https://www.ncbi.nlm.nih.gov/pmc/articles/PMC7087935/pdf/392_2020_Article_1626.pdf. *Retrieved 1 May, 2020.*
8. https://annals.org/aim/fullarticle/2762808/incubation-period-coronavirus-disease-2019-covid-19-from-publicly-reported. *Retrieved 1 May, 2020.*
9. Chang D, Lin M, Wei L, Xie L, Zhu G, Cruz CSD, Sharma L. Epidemiologic and clinical characteristics of novel coronavirus infections involving 13 patients outside Wuhan, China. JAMA 2020;323(11):1092–93.

10. https://www.medrxiv.org/content/10.1101/2020.02.24.20027268v1. *Retrieved 1 May, 2020.*

11. Montoya-Barthelemy A, Lee CD, Cundiff D, Smith E. COVID-19 and the Correctional Environment: The American Prison as a Focal Point for Public Health. *American Journal of Preventive Medicine* 2020.

12. https://www.medrxiv.org/content/10.1101/2020.02.24.20027268v1. *Retrieved 1 May, 2020.*

13. https://www.livemint.com/news/india/india-s-covid-19-doubling-rate-slower-mortality-rate-lower-than-us-italy-spain-uk-11588242585908.html. *Retrieved 1 May, 2020.*

14. https://www.who.int/news-room/commentaries/detail/modes-of-transmission-of-virus-causing-covid-19-implications-for-ipc-precaution-recommendations. *Retrieved 1 May, 2020.*

15. *"National Centre for Disease Control Directorate General of Health Services MoHFW, GOI, New Delhi"* https://ncdc.gov.in. *Retrieved 1 May, 2020.*

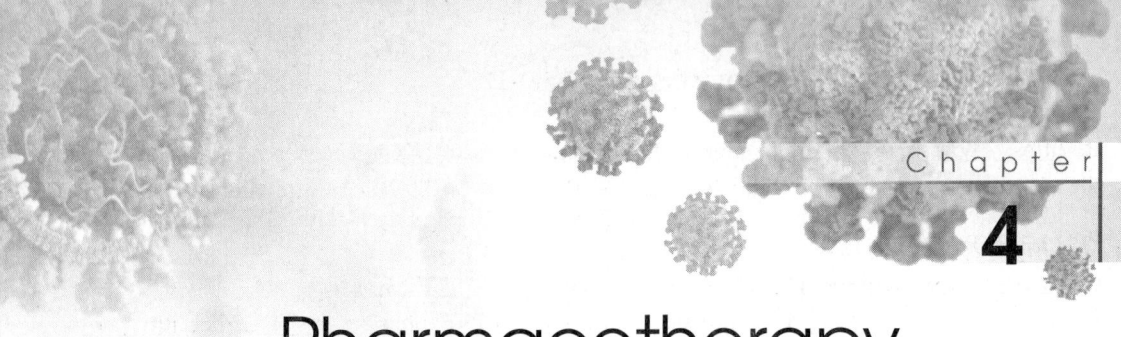

4

Pharmacotherapy

Amit Singh, Bisweswar Ojha, Bhairav Pathak

In general, antiviral drugs target various stages of replication like cell entry (antireceptor antibodies, fusion protein inhibitors), uncoating (ion channel blocker, capsid stabilizers), transcription of viral genome (inhibitor of viral DNA polymerase, RNA polymerase, reverse transcriptase, helicase, primase, or integrase), translation of viral proteins (interferons, antisense nucleotide, ribozymes, inhibitors of regulatory proteins), post-translational modification (protease inhibitors) and release inhibitors.

There are no specific drugs approved by the Food and Drug Administration (FDA) to treat the disease caused by the newly emergent SARS-CoV-2 virus (COVID-19). There are no clinical trial data supporting any prophylactic therapy. There are three classes of antiviral drugs under clinical trial for the efficacy and safety of drug against COVID-19. More than 300 active clinical trials are underway.

ANTIMICROBIAL DRUGS

RNA Polymerase Inhibitors

Remdesivir (RDV), an adenosine nucleotide analog, interferes viral RNA-dependent RNA polymerase. RDV was originally developed for the treatment of Ebola virus disease (EVD). It shows antiviral activities against several RNA viruses[1–3], including SARS-CoV and MERS-CoV.[4] RDV is having potent *in vitro* activity against several novel coronavirus (nCoVs), including SARS-CoV-2 with EC50 and EC90 values of 0.77 μM and 1.76 μM, respectively.[5] A few case reports support the use of RDV for SARS-CoV-2 infection.[6,7] At present, nine clinical trials are ongoing to evaluate the antiviral activity of RDV in patients with mild to moderate or severe COVID-19 (NCT04292899, NCT04292730, NCT04257656, NCT04252664, NCT04280705).

Favipiravir (FPV) is effective against a wide range of types and subtypes of influenza viruses, including strains resistant to existing anti-influenza drugs. The unique antiviral profiles will make FPV a potentially promising drug for specifically untreatable RNA viral infections. It has recently been demonstrated that, FPV (EC50 was 61.88 μmol/l) effectively inhibits the SARS-CoV-2 infection in Vero E6 cells[8] and *in vivo* studies are recommended to evaluate FPV.

Ribavirin, a guanine analogue, inhibits viral RNA-dependent RNA polymerase. Its activity against other nCoVs makes it a candidate for COVID-19 treatment. However, its *in vitro* activity against SARS-CoV was limited and required high concentrations to inhibit viral replication, necessitating high-dose and combination therapy.

Protease Inhibitors

CoVs replicase gene encodes two overlapping polyproteins, pp1a and pp1ab, required for viral replication and transcription.[9,10] The polyprotein is converted to functional polypeptides by protease (M^{pro}). **Lopinavir** is structurally similar to **ritonavir** but is 3- to 10-fold more potent against HIV-1. Lopinavir is available only in coformulation with low doses of ritonavir used as a CYP3A4 inhibitor. Lopinavir demonstrated *in vitro* activity against other novel coronaviruses via inhibition of 3-chymotrypsin-like protease. No published SARS-CoV-2 *in vitro* data exist for lopinavir or ritonavir. There are 22 ongoing clinical trials in progress for COVID-19.

Chloroquine and Hydroxychloroquine

They appear to block viral entry into cells by inhibiting glycosylation of host receptors, proteolytic processing, and endosomal acidification. These agents also have immunomodulatory effects through attenuation of cytokine production and inhibition of autophagy and lysosomal activity in host cells. Chloroquine inhibits SARS-CoV-2 *in vitro* with a half-maximal effective concentration (EC50) in the low micromolar range. Hydroxychloroquine has *in vitro* activity with a lower EC50 for SARS-CoV-2 compared with chloroquine after 24 hours of growth (hydroxychloroquine: EC50 = 6.14 μM and chloroquine: EC50 = 23.90 μM).[11]

Several anthelminthic drugs, **niclosamide, nitazoxanide** and **ivermectin** exhibited very potent antiviral activity against SARS-CoV-2.

Some other drugs like baricitinib, imatinib, dasatinib, and cyclosporine demonstrate *in vitro* activity against SARS-CoV-2.

Non-Specific (Anti-Inflammatory/Immunomodulators)

Interferons are cytokines that possess antiviral, immunomodulatory, and antiproliferative effects. These IFNs are synthesized by host cells in response to viral infections. Three major classes of human IFNs with significant antiviral activity currently are recognized: α, β, and γ. IFNs activate the Jak-STAT signal transduction pathway and lead to synthesis of over two dozen proteins that contribute to viral resistance mediated at different stages of viral penetration. High dose IFN treatment has antiviral effects against SARS-CoV and MERS-CoV *in vitro*.[12] Systemic interferon has been used to treat patients with SARS and MERS, although clinical effects are unclear. Multiple clinical trials are underway investigating the potential effect of IFN-α in COVID-19.

Anticytokine: IL-6 appears to be a key driver of this dysregulated inflammation based on early case series from China.[13] **Tocilizumab** and **sarilumab** are monoclonal antibodies against IL-6 receptor. Other monoclonal antibody or immune modulatory agents in clinical trials in China or available for expanded access in the US include **bevacizumab** (antivascular endothelial growth factor medication; NCT04275414), **fingolimod** (immune modulator approved for multiple sclerosis; NCT04280588), and **eculizumab** (antibody inhibiting terminal complement; NCT04288713).

Corticosteroids are anti-inflammatory drugs, which may provide benefit in acute lung injury and acute respiratory distress syndrome (ARDS). However, they can delay viral clearance and increased risk of secondary infection.

Another potential treatment for COVID-19 is the use of convalescent plasma or **hyperimmune immunoglobulins.** The antibodies from recovered patients' plasma may help with both free virus and infected cell immune clearance. Anecdotal reports or protocols for convalescent plasma have been reported as salvage therapy in SARS and MERS.

BCG vaccination has been reported to offer broad protection to respiratory infections. It was observed that countries without universal policies of BCG vaccination (Italy, Nederland, USA) have more incidence of COVID-19 compared to countries with universal and long-standing BCG policies.

REFERENCES

1. Siegel D, Hui HC, Doerffler E, et al. Discovery and Synthesis of a Phosphoramidate Prodrug of a Pyrrolo[2,1-f][triazin-4-amino] Adenine C-Nucleoside (GS-5734) for the Treatment of Ebola and Emerging Viruses. J Med Chem. 2017;60(5):1648-1661. doi:10.1021/acs.jmedchem.6b01594

2. Lo MK, Jordan R, Arvey A, et al. GS-5734 and its parent nucleoside analog inhibit Filo-, Pneumo-, and Paramyxoviruses. Scientific Reports 2017 Mar;7:43395. DOI: 10.1038/srep43395.

3. Warren TK, Jordan R, Lo MK, et al. Therapeutic efficacy of the small molecule GS-5734 against Ebola virus in rhesus monkeys [published correction appears in ACS Chem Biol. 2016 May 20;11(5):1463]. Nature 2016;531(7594):381–385. doi:10.1038/nature17180.

4. Agostini ML, Andres EL, Sims AC, et al. Coronavirus Susceptibility to the Antiviral Remdesivir (GS-5734) Is Mediated by the Viral Polymerase and the Proofreading Exoribonuclease. mBio 2018;9(2):e00221-18. Published 2018 Mar 6. doi:10.1128/mBio.00221–18.

5. Wang M, Cao R, Zhang L, et al. Remdesivir and chloroquine effectively inhibit the recently emerged novel coronavirus (2019-nCoV) *in vitro*. Cell Res 2020;30(3): 269-271.doi:10.1038/s41422020-0282-0

6. Holshue M L, De Bolt C, Lindquist S, et al; Washington State 2019-nCoV Case Investigation Team. First case of 2019 novel coronavirus in the United States. N Engl J Med 2020;382 (10):929-936. doi:10.1056/NEJMoa2001191

7. Kujawski SA, Wong K, Collins J P, et al. First 12 patients with coronavirus disease 2019 (COVID-19) in the United States. Med Rxiv. Preprint posted March 9, 2020.doi:10.1101/2020.03.09.20032896

8. Wang M, Cao R, Zhang L, et al. Remdesivir and chloroquine effectively inhibit the recently emerged novel coronavirus (2019-nCoV) *in vitro*. Cell Res 2020;30(3):269-271. doi:10.1038/s41422-020-0282-0.

9. Zhou P, Yang XL, Wang XG, et al. A pneumonia outbreak associated with a new coronavirus of probable bat origin. Nature 2020;579(7798):270-273. doi:10.1038/s41586-020-2012-7.

10. Wu F, Zhao S, Yu B, et al. A new coronavirus associated with human respiratory disease in China [published correction appears in Nature. 2020 Apr;580(7803):E7]. Nature 2020;579(7798):265–269. doi:10.1038/s41586-020-2008-3.

11. Yao X, Ye F, Zhang M, et al. *In vitro* antiviral activity and projection of optimized dosing design of hydroxychloroquine for the treatment of severe acute respiratory syndrome coronavirus 2 (SARS-CoV-2) [published online ahead of print, 2020 Mar 9]. Clin Infect Dis 2020;ciaa237. doi:10.1093/cid/ciaa237.

12. Cinatl J, Morgenstern B, Bauer G, Chandra P, Rabenau H, Doerr HW. Treatment of SARS with human interferons [published correction appears in Lancet. 2003 Aug 30;362(9385):748]. Lancet 2003;362(9380):293–294. doi:10.1016/s0140-6736(03)13973-6.

13. Zhou F, Yu T, Du R, et al. Clinical course and risk factors for mortality of adult in patients with COVID-19 in Wuhan, China: A retrospective cohort study. Lancet 2020;395 (10229):1054 –1062.doi: 10.1016/S0140-6736(20)30566–3.

Laboratory Investigations

Tuhina Banerjee, Arghya Das

Laboratory investigation for SARS-CoV-2 is an integral part of the strategic approach for containment of the COVID-19 pandemic. The currently available tests for laboratory diagnosis of COVID-19 are discussed in this chapter.

COLLECTION, STORAGE AND TRANSPORTATION OF SPECIMENS

The diagnostic strategy presently recommends testing of samples taken from the respiratory tract to assess for the presence of one or several nucleic acid targets specific to SARS-CoV-2. Although nasopharyngeal specimen is preferred over other swab-based specimens for SARS-CoV-2 testing, swab specimens collected from oropharynx, mid-turbinate, or anterior nares are also acceptable.[1,2] A flocked swab is considered ideal for specimens to enhance the collection and release of cellular material. Swabs with a plastic or aluminium shaft should be used. Substances like wood, cotton and calcium alginate may inhibit PCR-based molecular testing. Swabs containing these materials should be avoided for collection of specimens. Swab specimens need to be transferred immediately after collection into the universal viral transport medium (VTM) to preserve viral nucleic acid. Lower respiratory specimens, viz. sputum, endotracheal aspirate (ETA), and bronchoalveolar lavage (BAL) are more sensitive than the upper respiratory specimens.[3] But collection of these specimens specially ETA, BAL needs technical expertise and should only be done where needed (patients admitted in intensive care unit) and proper facilities are in place for collecting these specimens. Induction of the sputum is not recommended.[1] Whole blood specimens should be collected taking sterile precautions in vials without anticoagulant or serum separator tube for serological testing.[4] Two different blood specimens (acute and convalescent phase) should be collected for testing with a gap of 2–3 weeks between acute and convalescent stages. A detailed list of specimen types, collection materials, and storage, transport conditions for detection of SARS-CoV-2 is mentioned in Table 5.1.[5]

Precautions Adopted During Collection

Inadequate sample collection may result in a false-negative test. Airborne precaution needs to be adopted while collecting lower respiratory specimens because of possibility of generating aerosols during the procedure. Healthcare personnel collecting specimens

Table 5.1: Types of collection materials, transportation and storage of different specimens

Specimen	Collection materials	Transportation temperature	Storage temperature
Nasopharyngeal and oropharyngeal swab	Dacron or polyester flocked swabs dipped in VTM	4°C	≤5 days: 4°C >5 days:–70°C
Bronchoalveolar lavage	Sterile container with VTM	4°C	≤48 hours: 4°C >48 hours:–70°C
Tracheal aspirate, nasopharyngeal aspirator nasal wash	Sterile container with VTM	4°C	≤48 hours: 4°C >48 hours:–70°C
Sputum	Sterile container	4°C	≤48 hours: 4°C >48 hours:–70°C
Whole blood	Serum separator tubes/vials without anticoagulant	4°C	≤5 days: 4°C >5 days:–70°C

should wear personal protective equipment (PPE), viz. gown, head cover, eye protection (goggles or face shield), FFP2/N95 respirator (fit tested) and gloves. Wherever feasible, specimens should be collected in a negative pressure room. If not available, then specimens are collected in a room with the door closed and then the room should be left vacant for at least 30 minutes. Surfaces inside the room should be cleanly wiped with disinfectant wipes by a person wearing gloves, gown and surgical mask.[6]

All specimen containers should be properly labelled with permanent markers to avoid sample mismatching.

Storage of Specimens

Specimens can be preserved at 2–8°C for up to 48 hours after collection prior to testing. If further delay in testing of the specimen is anticipated, specimens should be stored at or less than 70°C.[6]

Transport of Specimens

Collected specimen in the container should be placed in the specimen collection bags and packaging/boxes with cold-packs or dry ice. Test order slip should be kept separate from the specimen container. If shipping of specimen is required for sending to any reference laboratory, specimen containers should be packed in accordance with the recent Dangerous Goods Regulations of the International Air Transport Association (IATA).[7]

LABORATORY-BASED INVESTIGATIONS

Laboratories performing tests for SARS-CoV-2 should adhere to the strict biosafety measures. A Biosafety Level 2 (BSL-2) containment facility with calibrated biosafety cabinet type 2A/2B is required for molecular testing of the specimens.[5] Isolation of SARS-CoV-2 virus in cell culture and initial characterization of viral agents recovered in cultures must be done in a BSL-3 laboratory.[8]

Laboratory-Based Nucleic Acid Amplification Test (NAAT)

The genetic heterogeneity of human coronaviruses (HCoVs) precludes the possibility of a single 'pan-HCoV' molecular test for new coronaviruses. The prompt effort of sequencing of the viral genome has enabled quick development of several molecular platforms which can detect SARS-CoV-2 targeting the snippets of the viral genome. *N* (nucleocapsid), *E* (envelope), *S* (spike protein) and *RdRP* (RNA-dependent RNA polymerase) genes are the mostly frequently targeted genes in the molecular assays.[5] The molecular assay recommended by the World Health Organization uses the primer-probe sets which target the SARS-CoV-2 *E and RdRP* genes. It differs from the assay developed by Centers for Disease Control and Prevention (CDC), USA, which uses PCR primer-probe sets targeting for two regions of the viral nucleocapsid gene (*N1* and *N2*). Both the assays are highly sensitive for SARS-CoV-2, with minimal cross-reactivity with other circulating strains of coronaviruses. To ensure adequate extraction of nucleic acids from the specimens, primer-probe targeting human *RNase P* gene has also been incorporated as internal extraction control in these assays.[9]

The laboratory-based molecular testing is primarily based on detection of unique sequences of viral RNA by NAAT such as real-time reverse-transcription polymerase chain reaction (rRT-PCR).[5] Although, the rRT-PCR is considered to be the current reference standard test where an 'undetected result' indicates the absence of SARS-CoV-2 in the clinical specimen, the sensitivity of the test may actually vary based on type and quality of specimen collected for testing. Any test result should be carefully correlated with patient's history and clinical presentation.[10]

Principle of rRT-PCR

The entire diagnostic protocol consists of extraction of RNA, reverse transcription of RNA to complementary DNA (cDNA) and subsequent amplification of the target sequence. Since PCR can only amplify dsDNA target sequences, single-stranded RNA targets need to be converted into cDNA sequence which can then be amplified by PCR. This process of reverse hybridization is carried out by the enzyme reverse transcriptase. To generate cDNA from template RNA using the enzyme reverse transcriptase, a primer is first annealed to the template. Specific primer sequences targeting the particular gene target are used in this process. Using these primers, reverse transcriptase synthesizes cDNA strand by adding complementary base pairs. The template RNA is then removed with the help of the enzyme RNase H leaving behind the newly generated single-stranded cDNA.

In the PCR process, the probe anneals to a specific target sequence located between the forward and reverse primers. During the extension phase of the PCR cycle, the 5' nuclease activity of Taq polymerase degrades the probe, causing the reporter dye to be separated from the quencher molecule, thus generating the fluorescent signal. More reporter dye molecules are cleaved from their respective probes with each cycle. This results in gradual increase in the fluorescence intensity. The intensity of fluorescent signal is monitored at each PCR cycle in real-time with the real-time PCR system.[11] The overall increase in fluorescence intensity is proportional to the amount of amplicon produced.

Precautions Followed during rRT-PCR

rRT-PCR is prone to accidental introduction of contaminating nucleic acid sequences or PCR product of previous amplifications reactions. The contamination may occur either in clinical specimen or the real-time reagents used in the amplification step.

Following measures need to be adopted and strictly followed to avoid contamination.[11]

- Workflow in the laboratory should follow a unidirectional pathway. The laboratories need to have separate areas designated for handling of nucleic acids, assay set-up, and running of the PCR.
- The expiry date of all the reagents must be checked before use. Mixing or substituting reagents from different lots from the same manufactures or from other manufacturers must be avoided.
- Single use powder-free gloves should be worn while performing different procedures inside the laboratory. Gloves need to be changed whenever contamination is suspected.
- There should be separate dedicated instruments (e.g. pipettes, microcentrifuges) and consumables (e.g. microcentrifuge tubes, pipette tips) for nucleic acid extraction and assay set-up.
- Aerosol barrier pipette tips should be used and changed between all manual liquid transfers.
- Reagent and reaction tubes should be kept capped or covered as much as possible.
- To ensure stability of the RNA, it should be maintained at cold temperature using ice or cold blocks during preparation and use.
- Enzyme master mix, primers, and probes (including aliquots) must be thawed and kept on cold block at all times during preparation and use.
- Pipettes, centrifuges and work-surfaces should be wiped and decontaminated with cleaning products such as "DNAZap™", "RNase AWAY®" or 10% bleach to minimize risk of nucleic acid contamination. Residual bleach should be finally wiped off with 70% ethanol.
- Used or unused reagents and human specimens should be disposed in accordance to the local or country-based regulations for biomedical waste management.

Workflow of rRT-PCR

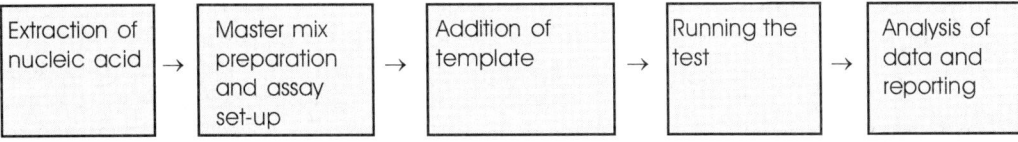

Extraction of nucleic acid → Master mix preparation and assay set-up → Addition of template → Running the test → Analysis of data and reporting

Extraction of nucleic acid: The specimens received for testing in the laboratory should initially be handled under BSL-3 conditions until the specimen or an aliquot is rendered non-infectious by lysis or another method.[12] Unpacking of the specimens should be done inside the designated biosafety cabinets (class II or higher). Compliance to good laboratory practices is essential while preparation of the specimens to minimize the risk of cross-contamination between samples, and the inadvertent introduction of nucleases into specimens during and after the extraction procedure. The performance of rRT-PCR hugely depends on the quality and quantity of the template nucleic acid extracted from clinical specimens. There is a wide variety of commercially available lysis buffers for nucleic acid extraction from different manufacturers (QIAGEN, Roche, bioMérieux). The concentration of inactivating agents in these lysis buffers has been found to be effective for inactivation of SARS-CoV-2.[11] The extraction procedure must follow the prescribed steps by the manufacturer.

Preparation of master mix and assay set-up: Master mix is prepared inside clean hood in the designated reagent set-up room. The reagents, rRT-PCR buffer, enzyme, and primer/probes are placed on ice or cold-block. The number of reactions (N) to set up per assay is first determined taking into consideration the number of specimens to be tested, negative, positive, and extraction controls. For each primer/probe set, the amount of each reagent to be added for each reaction mixture is calculated following the manufacturer's guidelines. The reagents are dispensed in the microcentrifuge tube with pipette. After addition, the reagents are gently mixed by pipetting up and down. Vortexing of the reaction mixtures is avoided. Prior to proceeding to the nucleic acid template addition room, the negative control/negative template control (NTC) reaction set up should be completed in the assay preparation area.[11]

Nucleic acid template addition: Addition of template nucleic acids to the reaction mixture in the assay set-up must be done very carefully avoiding any chance of contaminating the assay set-up. Gloves need to be often changed when necessary to avoid cross-contamination. The positive template control/positive control (PC) must be added after all the specimens have been added in their respective wells and securely capped.[11]

Running of assay in the RT-PCR system: After inserting the assay plate inside the real-time PCR instrument, the test is run according to the protocol in the installed software. Care should be taken at this stage to properly label each assay well or tube's position in the software by adding patients' identifiers, specimen number, date.

Data analysis: Amplification of human *RNase P* gene must be checked to ensure specimen quality and extraction. Fluorescence curves in the *RNase P* reaction which cross the threshold limit must be present for all clinical specimens. Failure to detect *RNase P* in any clinical specimen would indicate:

- Improper extraction of nucleic acid from clinical materials resulting in loss of RNA and/or RNA degradation.
- Absence of sufficient human cellular material due to poor collection or loss of specimen integrity.
- Improper assay set up and execution.
- Reagent or equipment malfunction.

A negative *RNase P* signal does not preclude the presence of SARS-CoV-2 RNA in a clinical specimen. A positive result for SARS-CoV-2 specific gene markers should be considered valid even in the absence of *RNase P* signal which may sometimes occur, if the quantity of human cells is less in the original clinical specimen. If both SARS-CoV-2 specific gene marker and *RNase P* signals are absent for a particular reaction, the result should be considered invalid for the specimen. In such cases, the extraction procedure and test process should be repeated with residual specimen, if any. If all markers remain negative even after retesting, the result is reported as invalid and fresh specimen must be collected and processed for testing.[11]

Quality Control and Quality Assurance

Quality control (QC) standards must be met as per the local, country level accreditation requirements for the laboratories performing rRT-PCR for SARS-CoV-2. The QC measures are applied to ensure the performance of the assay and the reagents.[11]

Following are the types of external controls must be included in each assay run.

1. **No template control (NTC):** Nuclease-free water is used as NTC in the rRT-PCR. The intensity fluorescent signal from all primer and probe sets with NTC should not cross the threshold limit. If a fluorescent signal curve that crosses the cycle threshold in any of the reaction set with NTC is detected, possibility of contamination during specimen extraction and/or plate set-up must be considered. The entire cycle run is invalidated and specimens are processed again.
2. **Positive control (PC):** The PC consists of SARS-CoV-2 RNA transcribed *in vitro*. Multiple freeze-thaw cycle for this control must be avoided to maintain the integrity of the control RNA material. Multiple aliquots should be prepared after reconstitution of the dried reagent, stored at –80°C and only one aliquot is thawed for each batch of experiments. The positive control should yield a positive result with the primer and probe sets in the test run.
3. **Extraction control/human specimen control (HSC):** HSC consists of material containing non-infectious human cells. It serves as nucleic acid extraction procedural control to validate the integrity of extraction reagents and also to demonstrate recovery of RNA from clinical specimens. The extraction control should be included in each batch of specimens and processed through the nucleic acid extraction protocol.

Whole Genome Sequencing

Next-generation sequencing (NGS) helps in differentiating SARS-CoV-2 from other circulating HCoVs. NGS is a high-throughput method to sequence nucleic acids. Unlike the classic Sanger sequencing method, NGS provides millions to billions copies of short nucleotide sequences within a few hours at relatively lower costs. As soon as a reference sequence becomes available, NGS can help in sequencing of genetic material obtained from clinical specimen, then align the new sequence to the reference to detect mutations or single nucleotide polymorphisms (SNPs) annotating the nucleotide differences. It is the timely effort of the scientists working with NGS which has led to the early discovery of the novel SARS-CoV-2. The whole genome sequencing with NGS also helps to detect the genetic relatedness of different strains of SARS-CoV-2; credit goes to the sequencing redundancy, quasispecies analysis.[13]

Point of Care Molecular Diagnostics

These are user friendly, labour non-intensive molecular diagnostic platforms with less turnaround time. Xpert Xpress SARS-CoV-2 (Cepheid), ID NOW™ COVID-19 (Abbott Laboratories), Accula SARS-CoV-2 Test (Mesa Biotech), ePlex SARS-CoV-2 (GenMark

Diagnostics Inc.) are the FDA (Food and Drug Administration) authorized molecular assays for use outside the laboratory by non-laboratory personnel for detection of SARS-CoV-2.[14]

Xpert Xpress SARS-CoV-2

This cartridge-based nucleic acid amplification test (CBNAAT) is developed by Cephid for qualitative detection of SARS-CoV-2 in either nasopharyngeal, nasal, or mid-turbinate swab and/or nasal wash/aspirate specimens collected from individuals suspected of COVID-19. The newly developed Xpert Xpress SARS-CoV-2 cartridge can be used on Cepheid's GeneXpert® Systems which have a worldwide footprint of more than 23,000 placements and have earlier revolutionized the diagnosis of tuberculosis.

The single-use disposable cartridges hold the reagents which are required for RT-PCR. Possibility of cross-contamination between clinical specimens is minimized owing to self-contained design of the cartridges. Besides the reagents for the detection of RNA from SARS-CoV-2, the cartridge also contains the sample processing control (SPC) and the probe check control (PCC). SPC ensures adequate processing of the sample, effectiveness of the reagents, appropriate temperature and also monitors for the presence of potential inhibitor(s) in the RT-PCR reaction. The PCC ensures reagent rehydration, PCR tube filling, monitors for probe integrity and dye stability and also confirms the presence of all reaction components inside the cartridge.[15]

The nasopharyngeal, nasal, or mid-turbinate swab specimen and/or nasal wash/aspirate specimen is collected and placed into a viral transport tube containing 3 ml transport medium. The specimen is briefly mixed by rapidly inverting the collection tube 5 times. Using the supplied transfer pipette, the sample is transferred to the sample chamber of the Xpert Xpress SARS-CoV-2 cartridge. The GeneXpert cartridge is loaded onto the GeneXpert Instrument System platform, which performs hands-off, automated sample processing, and real-time RT-PCR for detection of viral RNA.

The test can rapidly detect of the coronavirus SARS-CoV-2 in approximately 45 minutes and requires less than a minute of hands on time for specimen preparation.[16] The collected specimen into the tube containing transport medium is briefly mixed by rapidly inverting the collection tube 4–5 times. The sample is then transferred to the sample chamber of the cartridge with the disposable transfer pipette. The GeneXpert cartridge is loaded onto the GeneXpert System where hands-off, automated sample processing, and real-time RT-PCR for detection of viral RNA are performed. The results are interpreted by the GeneXpert System itself based on the amplification of two gene targets (N2 and E) and are displayed in the 'View Results' window of the software (Table 5.2).

Table 5.2: Reporting of Xpert Xpress SARS-CoV-2 testing

Result	N2	E	SPC
SARS-CoV-2 positive	+	+/–	+/–
SARS-CoV-2 presumptive POS	–	+	+/–
SARS-CoV-2 negative	–	–	+
Invalid	–	–	–

A positive test result does not rule out co-infection with other viruses or bacteria and a negative result does not preclude the presence of SARS-CoV-2. Thus, this should not be used as a standalone test to decide for treatment or management of the COVID-19 patients. As with any molecular test, the major limitation of Xpress SARS-CoV-2 is that the mutations within the target regions can affect primer and/or probe binding resulting in failure to detect the presence of virus. Moreover, the performance of the Xpert Xpress SARS-CoV-2 test has only been established in nasopharyngeal swab and nasal wash/aspirate specimens. Although nasal swabs and mid-turbinate swabs are considered acceptable specimen, the performance of Xpert Xpress SARS-CoV-2 with these and all other types of specimens has not been assessed.[15]

ID NOW™ COVID-19

The ID NOW™ COVID-19 assay for use on the ID NOW (Abbott Laboratories) platform has received emergency use authorization (EUA) from US FDA. The molecular target in this assay is the RdRP gene of SARS-CoV-2 virus. This has got several advantages like storage of reagents at room temperature, direct processing of clinical specimens like nasopharyngeal and oropharyngeal swabs, availability of positive results in as little as 5 minutes and negative results in 13 minutes.[17]

Accula SARS-CoV-2

The Accula SARS-CoV-2 (Mesa Biotech) is another rapid point of care diagnostic testing that has received FDA EUA. This platform utilizes the principle of PCR and lateral flow technology for the qualitative, visual detection of the coronavirus SARS-CoV-2 in approximately 30 minutes. The collected throat swab or nasal specimens are first solubilized in SARS-CoV-2 buffer. An aliquot from the buffer is then dispensed in Accula SARS-CoV-2 test cassette which contains enzymes, OscAR™ reagents, internal process positive and negative controls and a detection strip necessary for the 4 steps in the assay, viz. lysis of the virus, reverse transcription of viral RNA to cDNA, nucleic acid amplification, and detection.[18]

Truenat™ Beta CoV Test

The Indian Council of Medical Research (ICMR) has validated Truenat™ beta CoV test on Truenat™ workstation (Molbio Diagnostics) has recommended the test for screening of SARS-CoV-2.[19] A positive Truenat™ beta CoV test result generated in the Truenat laboratory should be confirmed with the real-time RT-PCR test results performed in the concerned/mapped ICMR registered laboratory for COVID-19 real-time RT-PCR testing.

Clustered Regularly Interspersed Short Palindromic Repeats (CRISPR) Based Molecular Diagnostics

This highly sensitive, specific approach is in the diagnostic pipeline under evaluation as potential point of care test, at the time of writing this chapter. One such technique, CRISPR-based SHERLOCK (Specific High Sensitivity Enzymatic Reporter UnLOCKing) by Sherlock Biosciences Inc uses synthetic SARS-CoV-2 RNA fragments detecting the viral target sequences as low as 10–100 copies per microliter in clinical specimens. The result can be obtained in less than one hour using dipstick without requiring sophisticated instruments.[20]

SEROLOGICAL TESTS

Serological tests such as enzyme-linked immunosorbent assay (ELISA), immuno-chromatographic test (lateral flow assays), etc. are less complex than molecular tests those are aimed to detect specific antibodies (IgM, IgG) from clinical specimens like serum or whole blood. As SARS-CoV-2 is a new virus, specific antibodies to the virus are absent in the broader population who have not been exposed to the virus.[21] Following any infection, antibodies take time (days to weeks) to appear in the blood. Thus, the utility of serological tests in diagnosis of acute infections can be limited because the viral shedding and transmission risk seem to be highest around the time of onset of symptoms when antibodies are usually not detectable in blood (Fig. 5.1). So, a negative serological test does not obviate the need of confirmatory molecular tests like rRT-PCR. On the other hand, a positive result may be due to either ongoing or the past infection. There is also the possibility of a positive result owing to the cross-reactivity of the antibodies against other circulatory HCoVs to SARS-CoV-2 coronavirus antigens.[22] A rise in antibody level between acute and convalescent phase sera may suggest a recent infection.[21] Moreover, the serologic assays might be more relevant in situations where patients present late with complications of the disease and viral shedding has decreased below the detection of rRT-PCR making the aetiological diagnosis of COVID-19 difficult.[23]

Days of Infection

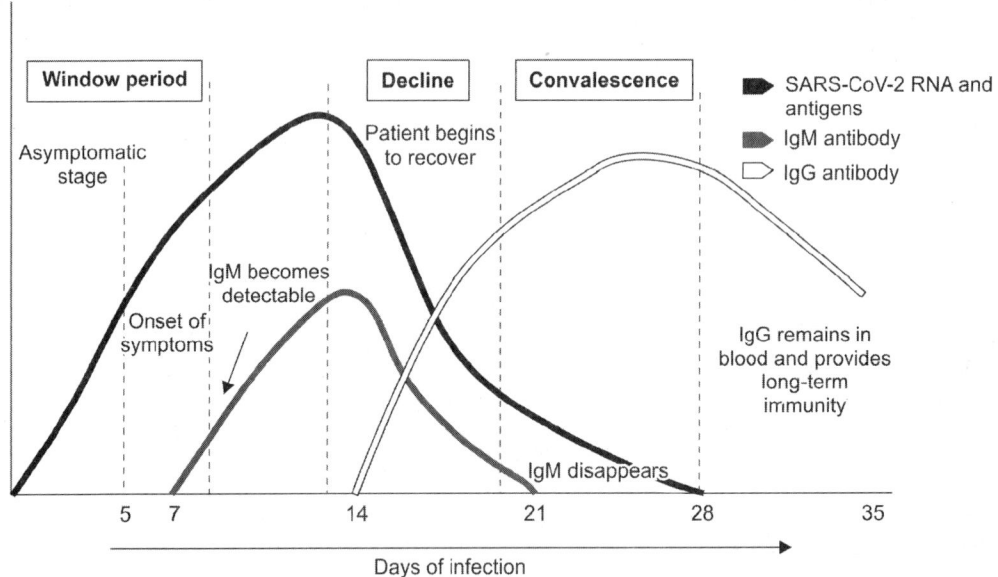

Fig. 5.1: Viral and serological markers in different stages of SARS-CoV-2 infection (*Image courtesy: Dr Rituparna Dasgupta, RIMS, Ranchi*)

Additionally, these serological tests would be particularly useful in vaccine trial verifying the effectiveness of the vaccines, or can be used in contact tracing in ongoing surveillance as well as in seroepidemiological studies to know the natural history of the disease.[24]

Table 5.3: Clinical interpretation of viral and serological markers in different stages of SARS-CoV-2 infection

Investigations			Stage of infection/interpretation
RT-PCR	Serological test		
Viral RNA	IgM	IgG	
+	–	–	Window period
+	+	–	Early stage of symptomatic infection
+	+	+	Active stage of symptomatic infection
+	–	+	Late stage of infection/recurrence
–	–	+	Recovery/past infection
–	+	+	Late stage of infection/false negative molecular test/cross-reactivity with non-SARS-CoV-2 coronaviruses

ISOLATION OF VIRUS IN CELL LINE

Routinely isolation of human coronaviruses (HCoV) is not performed in laboratory for diagnosis owing to long turnaround time, labour intensiveness, and lack of permissive cell lines and commercially available antisera for confirmation of viral growth in cell lines.[9] Although severe acute respiratory syndrome coronavirus (SARS-CoV) and Middle East respiratory syndrome coronavirus (MERS-CoV) and SARS-CoV-2 can grow in primary monkey cells and cell lines such as Vero and LLCMK2, cell culture should be avoided in routine diagnostic laboratories for biosafety concerns. However, virus isolation in cell cultures is crucial to obtain for characterization viruses and also supports the development of vaccines and testing of potential therapeutic agents.[9]

Both nasopharyngeal and oropharyngeal swab specimens have been used for isolation of SARS-CoV-2 using Vero E6, Vero CCL-81, HUH 7.0, 293T, A549, and EFKB3 cells suspended in Dulbecco minimal essential medium (DMEM) supplemented with heat-inactivated fetal bovine serum (5% or 10%) and penicillin/streptomycin and amphotericin B. After trypsinization, the cell suspension with pipette is directly added with the clinical specimen dilutions in the wells of tissue culture plate and mixed gently. The inoculated cultures should be incubated at 37°C in humidified 5% CO_2 atmosphere till cytopathic effect (CPE) is observed.[25] Standard plaque assays which are based on the same principle as for SARS-CoV and Middle East respiratory syndrome coronavirus (MERS-CoV) can be used for SARS-CoV-2.[26,27] After CPE has been observed, total nucleic acid extraction should be performed from scraped cell monolayers for confirmatory molecular testing and sequencing.[25]

DETECTION OF VIRAL ANTIGENS

Rapid antigen detection tests are low-cost detections systems providing quicker test results but are plagued by questionable poor sensitivity for detection of HCoVs.[9] Timing of specimen collection, when viral titres are high, is crucial and may improve the diagnostic yield of these tests.[28] Simple and rapid fluorescence immunochromatographic assay has been developed for detecting SARS-CoV-2 nucleocapsid protein in nasopharyngeal swab.[29] Other monoclonal antibodies specifically against SARS-CoV-2 are under development, which might provide the opportunity for highly sensitive and specific rapid antigen detection test in near future.[9]

ANCILLARY LABORATORY TESTS

The role of clinical laboratories extends beyond the aetiological diagnosis of the COVID-19 patients. Biochemical monitoring of COVID-19 patients is a critical aspect for assessment of disease severity, progression as well as for treatment monitoring. Several common parameters implicated in unfavourable outcome in COVID-19 patients are included in Table 5.4.

Table 5.4: Laboratory test parameters and underlying clinicopathological condition

Laboratory test	Abnormalities observed in adult COVID-19 patients with unfavourable outcome	Underlying clinicopathological condition
Complete blood count	Increased white blood cells (WBCs)	Superadded bacterial infection
	Increased neutrophil count	Superadded bacterial infection
	Decreased lymphocyte count	Immunological hyporesponsiveness to the virus
	Decreased platelet count	Disseminated intravascular coagulopathy
Prothrombin time (PT)	Increased	Disseminated intravascular coagulopathy
D-dimer	Increased	Disseminated intravascular coagulopathy
Total bilirubin	Increased	Liver injury
Alanine aminotransferase (ALT)/SGPT	Increased	Liver injury
Aspartate aminotransferase (AST)/SGOT	Increased	Liver injury
Albumin	Decreased	Impaired liver function
Lactate dehydrogenase (LDH)	Increased	Lung injury
Creatinine	Increased	Renal injury
Cardiac troponin	Increased	Cardiac injury
Procalcitonin (PCT)	Increased	Superadded bacterial infection
C-reactive protein (CRP)	Increased	Severe viral infection/viraemia
Ferritin	Increased	Severe inflammation
Cytokines (IL-6)	Increased	Cytokine storm

The most common laboratory features frequently reported in patients with COVID-19 are decreased albumin, increased C-reactive protein (CRP), and increased lactate dehydrogenase levels (LDH), and lymphopenia.[30] There are other biomarkers which have also been reported, viz. increased erythrocyte sedimentation rates; elevated aspartate aminotransferase, alanine aminotransferase, bilirubin, creatinine levels, and leukopenia, leucocytosis.[31-33] It needs to be clearly understood that these deranged biochemical parameters are not exclusive for COVID-19 and can also be found in different organ dysfunction or pathologies due to other infection or morbidities.

In addition, cytokines can be used as a biomarker to assess severe inflammatory response particularly the cytokine storm/macrophage activation syndrome (MAS). Hyperactive and overzealous immune response is mostly confined to the lung parenchyma or adjacent bronchoalveolar lymphoid tissue and leads to the development of ARDS. Sustained increase in interleukin levels, IL-6 in particular, has been linked to increased mortality in ARDS and may serve as a potential prognostic biomarker.[34] However, these biomarkers need to be rigorously evaluated before they can be used to pragmatically predict the clinical course of COVID-19 or used as surrogate markers for cure following successful treatment in the diseased patients.

REFERENCES

1. Centers for Disease Control and Prevention. Interim Guidelines for Collecting, Handling, and Testing Clinical Specimens from Persons for Coronavirus Disease 2019 (COVID-19). Atlanta, Georgia: Centers for Disease Control and Prevention; 2020.
   Available from www.cdc.gov/coronavirus/2019-nCoV/lab/guidelines-clinical-specimens.html [Accessed April 30, 2020].

2. Zou L, Ruan F, Huang M, et al. SARS-CoV-2 Viral Load in Upper Respiratory Specimens of Infected Patients. N Engl J Med 2020 Mar 19;382(12):1177–79.

3. Wang W, Xu Y, Gao R, et al. Detection of SARS-CoV-2 in different types of clinical specimens. JAMA 2020 Mar 11.

4. Department of Pathology and Laboratory Medicine. School of Medicine. University of California. Specimen Requirements/Containers. Irvine, CA: University of California.
   Available from http://www.pathology.uci.edu/services/specimen-containers.asp
   [Accessed April 30, 2020].

5. World Health Organization. Laboratory testing for coronavirus disease 2019 (COVID-19) in suspected human cases. Interim guidance. World Health Organization; 2020. Available from https://apps.who.int/iris/bitstream/handle/10665/331329/WHO-COVID-19-laboratory-2020.4-eng.pdf?sequence=1 and isAllowed=y [Accessed April 30, 2020].

6. Public Health Laboratory Network. Department of Health. Australian Government. PHLN guidance on laboratory testing for SARS-CoV-2 (the virus that causes COVID-19). Available from https://www.health.gov.au/sites/default/files/documents/2020/03/phln-guidance-on-laboratory-testing-for-sars-cov-2-the-virus-that-causes-covid-19.pdf [Accessed April 30, 2020].

7. International Air Transport Association. IATA Dangerous Goods Regulations (DGR). Available from https://www.iata.org/en/programs/cargo/dgr [Accessed April 30, 2020].

8. Centers for Disease Control and Prevention. Interim Laboratory Biosafety Guidelines for Handling and Processing Specimens Associated with Coronavirus Disease 2019 (COVID-19). Atlanta, Georgia: Centers for Disease Control and Prevention; 2020. Available from

https://www.cdc.gov/coronavirus/2019-nCoV/lab/lab-biosafety-guidelines.html [Accessed April 30, 2020].

9. Cheng MP, Papenburg J, Desjardins M, et al. Diagnostic Testing for Severe Acute Respiratory Syndrome-Related Coronavirus-2: A Narrative Review. Ann Intern Med. 2020 Apr 13.

10. Mayo Clinic Laboratories. Severe Acute Respiratory Syndrome Coronavirus 2 (SARS-CoV-2) RNA, Varies. Rochester, Minnesota: Mayo Clinic. Available from https://www.mayocliniclabs. com/test-catalog/Clinical+and+Interpretive/608934 [Accessed April 30, 2020].

11. Centers for Disease Control and Prevention. CDC 2019-Novel Coronavirus (2019-nCoV) Real-Time RT-PCR Diagnostic Panel. Atlanta, Georgia: Centers for Disease Control and Prevention; 2020. Available from https://www.fda.gov/media/134922/download [Accessed April 30, 2020].

12. Loeffelholz MJ, Tang YW. Laboratory diagnosis of emerging human coronavirus infections—the state of the art. Emerg Microbes Infect. 2020 Dec;9(1):747–756.

13. Campbell M. Further analysis of SARS-CoV-2 genome suggests it is stable. Technology Networks. Apr 07, 2020. Available from https://www.technologynetworks.com/genomics/blog/further-analysis-of-sars-cov-2-genome-suggests-it-is-stable-333162 [Accessed April 30, 2020].

14. Rosenthal M, Bronstein D. FDA Clears a Path for 5 Rapid SARS-CoV-2 Tests. Clinical Oncology News. April 8, 2020. Available from https://www.clinicaloncology.com/COVID-19/Article/04–20/FDA-Clears-a-Path-for-5-Rapid-SARS-CoV-2-Tests/57881 [Accessed April 30, 2020].

15. Cepheid. Xpert® Xpress SARS-CoV-2. Instructions for Use For Use Under an Emergency Use Authorization (EUA) Only. Sunnyvale, CA: Cepheid; 2020. Available from https://www.fda.gov/media/136314/download [Accessed April 30, 2020].

16. Cepheid. Xpert® Xpress SARS-CoV-2. Sunnyvale, CA: Cepheid; 2020. Available from https://www.cepheid.com/coronavirus [Accessed April 30, 2020].

17. Abbott. ID NOW™ COVID-19. Available from https://www.alere.com/en/home/product-details/id-now-covid-19.html [Accessed April 30, 2020].

18. Mesabiotech. Accula™ SARS-Cov-2 Test. San Diego, CA: Mesa Biotech, INC; 2020. Available from https://www.fda.gov/media/136355/download [Accessed April 30, 2020].

19. Indian Council of Medical Research. Department of Health Research. Guidance on the use of Truenat™ beta CoV. Available from https://icmr.nic.in/sites/default/files/upload_documents/Guidance_TrueNat_14042020.pdf [Accessed April 30, 2020].

20. Zhang F, Abudayyeh OO, Gootenberg JS. A protocol for detection of COVID-19 using CRISPR diagnostics. Available from https://www.broadinstitute.org/files/publications/special/COVID-19%20detection%20(updated).pdf [Accessed April 30, 2020].

21. World Health Organization. Emergencies preparedness, response. Use of laboratory methods for SARS diagnosis. World Health Organization; 2020. Available from https://www.who.int/csr/sars/labmethods/en/ [Accessed April 30, 2020].

22. Patrick DM, Petric M, Skowronski DM, et al. An outbreak of human coronavirus OC43 infection and serological cross-reactivity with SARS coronavirus. Can J Infect Dis Med Microbiol 2006;17:330–06.

23. To KK, Tsang OT, Leung WS, et al. Temporal profiles of viral load in posterior oropharyngeal saliva samples and serum antibody responses during infection by SARS-CoV-2: an observational cohort study. Lancet Infect Dis 2020.

24. US Food & Drug Administration. FAQs on Diagnostic Testing for SARS-CoV-2. Available from https://www.fda.gov/medical-devices/emergency-situations-medical-devices/faqs-diagnostic-testing-sars-cov-2 [Accessed April 30, 2020].

25. Harcourt J, Tamin A, Lu X, et al. Severe acute respiratory syndrome coronavirus 2 from patient with 2019 novel coronavirus disease, United States. Emerging Infectious Diseases 2020 Mar 11;26(6).

26. Sims AC, Tilton SC, Menachery VD, et al. Release of severe acute respiratory syndrome coronavirus nuclear import block enhances host transcription in human lung cells. J Virol. 2013;87:3885–3902.

27. Josset L, Menachery VD, Gralinski LE, et al. Cell host response to infection with novel human coronavirus EMC predicts potential antivirals and important differences with SARS coronavirus. MBio. 2013;4:e00165–213.

28. Bruning AHL, Aatola H, Toivola H, et al. Rapid detection and monitoring of human coronavirus infections. New Microbes New Infect. 2018;24:52–55.

29. Diao B, Wen K, Chen J, et al. Diagnosis of acute respiratory syndrome coronavirus 2 infection by detection of nucleocapsid protein. Med Rxiv. 2020 Jan 1.

30. Rodriguez-Morales AJ, Cardona-Ospina JA, Gutie´ rrez-Ocampo E, et al. Latin American Network of Coronavirus Disease 2019, COVID-19 Research (LANCOVID-19). Electronic address: https://www.lancovid.org. Clinical, laboratory and imaging features of COVID-19: a systematic review and meta-analysis. Travel Med Infect Dis. 2020:101623.

31. Chen L, Liu HG, Liu W, et al. Analysis of clinical features of 29 patients with 2019 novel coronavirus pneumonia. Zhonghua Jie He He Hu Xi Za Zhi 2020;43:203–08.

32. Chen N, Zhou M, Dong X, et al. Epidemiological and clinical characteristics of 99 cases of 2019 novel coronavirus pneumonia in Wuhan, China: a descriptive study. Lancet 2020;395:507–13.

33. Huang C, Wang Y, Li X, et al. Clinical features of patients infected with 2019 novel coronavirus in Wuhan, China. Lancet 2020;395:497–506.

34. McGonagle D, Sharif K, O'Regan A, Bridgewood C. The Role of Cytokines including Interleukin-6 in COVID-19 induced Pneumonia and Macrophage Activation Syndrome-Like Disease. Autoimmun Rev. 2020 Apr 3:102537.

Clinical Presentation

Anish K Saha, Deepak K Gautam

The present pandemic COVID-19 caused by a novel virus SARS-CoV-2 is ongoing. Its clinical manifestations are unfolding each day. Describing its clinical presentations may not be appropriate at this point of time. Only after multicentric data from different countries accrue and get compiled, could it be feasible to give a precise description of its myriad presentations. However, this being a viral illness, the usual set of symptoms termed collectively as coryza is likely to be present. The portal of entry is through the respiratory droplets or a fomite containing the same. This is similar to any other viral infection where the portal of entry is the respiratory tract.

Coryza consists of sneezing, coughing, runny nose, nasal congestion, pain in throat, fever, headache and reddish or itchy conjunctiva.

This would not be irrelevant to make a note here that coryza may not be stated as a complaint by a fair number of patients. This is due to the fact that sometimes it is very mild. It can be limited to occasional sneezes off and on. This can be non-specifically attributed to a few other disease states like allergic rhinitis, vasomotor rhinitis or a bacterial infection of the respiratory tract causing inflammation of the nasopharynx, nasal epithelium, nasal turbinate or the nasal septa.

The spectrum of remaining symptoms is wide and they range from mild to severe. Most of the infected individuals develop only mild to moderate symptoms and recover on their own. Here lies the importance of physical distancing, sneezing-coughing manners and avoiding contact with a potential fomite, e.g. the door handles at a common entrance.

Differential Diagnosis

There are a few differential diagnoses worth keeping in mind while assessing a suspect. These are: Common cold caused by rhinoviruses, coronaviruses other than SARS-CoV-2, adenovirus, respiratory syncytial virus, influenza and parainfluenza virus and H1N1 (swine) flu. All these present with a common symptom—cluster of coryza in majority of the patients.

Incubation period, i.e. the duration from exposure to onset of first symptom ranges from 2 to 14 days[1] with mean of 5–6 days.

COVID-19 Suspect

People with likelihood of exposure and having these symptoms[1] are considered as suspects of COVID-19:
- Cough
- Shortness of breath or difficulty breathing

Or at least two of these symptoms:[2, 4]
- Fever
- Chills
- Rigors
- Severe fatigue or prostration
- Myalgia
- Headache
- Sore throat
- Diarrhoea
- New onset loss of taste[3,7] (dysgeusia) and new onset loss of smell[3,7] (anosmia).

   A study published in the journal *International Forum of Allergy and Rhinology*, quotes that "if you have smell and taste loss, you are more than 10 times likely to have COVID-19 infection than any other infection". Dysgeusia and anosmia when present are associated with milder form of the disease.[3,7] In absence of complications, these symptoms are rapidly reversible with full recovery within 2–4 weeks.

Dermatological Findings

Dermatological findings in patients with COVID-19 are not well characterized. Reddish-purple nodules on the distal digits resembling *pernio* or chilblains have been described. They are seen mainly in children and young adults with confirmed or suspected COVID-19. Although an association has not been clearly established, some are calling this finding 'COVID toes' (Fig. 6.1). These lesions resemble acral gangrene similar to the one seen in cases associated with Raynaud's phenomenon. Observed COVID-associated skin patterns are:[5]

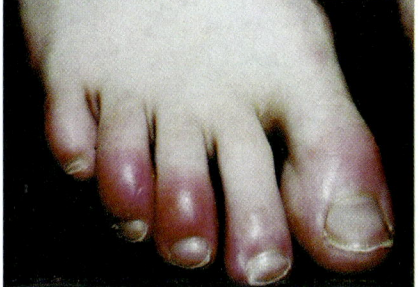

- Maculopapular eruptions (47%)
- Acral erythema with vesicles or pustules; so-called 'pseudo-chilblains' (19%)
- Urticaria (19%)
- Vesicular (chickenpox-like) eruptions (9%)
- Livedo or necrosis (6%)

Most Common Symptoms

Out of all the symptoms listed above, the set of most common ones are fever, dry cough and fatigue.[1–4]

Fig. 6.1: 'COVID toe' (*Courtesy:* Medscape; *source:* Wikimedia Commons)

Frequency of Symptoms

In a study on 138 patients, hospitalized with COVID-19 in Wuhan, the most common clinical features at the onset of illness were:[2]

- Fever in 99%
- Fatigue in 70%
- Dry cough in 59%
- Anorexia in 40%
- Myalgias in 35%
- Dyspnoea in 31%
- Sputum production in 27%

Children constitute only a small proportion of patients affected by this illness. COVID-19 in children presents with similar symptoms as that of adult but the course is usually milder than adults and the outcome much better with recovery in 1–2 weeks.

Symptoms Warranting Emergency Medical Help

The symptoms warranting emergency medical help are:[1,2]

- Breathlessness
- Persistent pain or pressure in the chest
- New onset confusion or inability to arouse
- Bluish lips or face
- Inability to speak and inability to move

Asymptomatic Infections

Asymptomatic infections are not uncommon. It is important to understand that in a herd of 619 passengers in a cruise ship, nearly half of the people who tested positive for SARS-CoV-2 were completely asymptomatic. So these are the subjects who disseminate the disease in absence of adequate physical distancing and sanitization.

Psychiatric Disorders

It is relevant to mention that the pandemic has resulted into anxiety and various phobias in masses. A number of patients who turn out to be negative on testing have symptoms due to this hypochondriasis. In the light of the reviews of past viral epidemics associated with neuropsychiatric symptoms such as demyelination, encephalopathy and neuromuscular dysfunction as well as mood instability and psychosis, the same cannot be ruled out in case of COVID-19. The disease is associated with multiple psychiatric issues not only in the patients but also in the clinicians who care for these patients.

Clinicians

In a cross-sectional study on more than 1,200 subjects using self-reporting instruments to assess physicians and nurses in China, the prevalence of moderate to severe psychiatric symptoms were:[6]

- Anxiety – 12%
- Depression – 15%
- Insomnia – 8%
- Traumatic distress – 35%

Patients with COVID-19

Self-reported stress[6] was greater among the infected patients than controls, as were negative psychological effects such as impaired sleep, dysphoria, lack of concentration and impaired judgment. However, majority of the patients and controls also reported positive psychological effects such as awareness of hygiene, physical state, and current affairs.

Patients with Existing Psychiatric Illnesses

Patients with anxiety and depression may be susceptible to the continuous media reporting about the pandemic and the stakes surrounding its consequences.[6] Moreover, the psychological effects of quarantine can be negative, including anger, confusion and symptoms of PTSD, and these effects may be long-lasting. Patients with serious mental illness, such as schizophrenia, are most susceptible to this pandemic. In addition, psychiatric illnesses that occur during the pandemic may arise from psychosocial factors such as:

- Frequency and extent of exposure to COVID-19 infected individuals
- Fear of infecting other members of the family
- Lack of access to testing and medical facilities
- Physical distancing, home confinement and quarantine
- Inconsistent messages and instructions regarding public health measures such as wearing face masks
- Hectic work schedules
- Financial hardships and insecurity
- Shortages of available resources (e.g. foods, paper products and PPE)
- Diminished personal liberty

As per the retrospective studies of the 2003 severe SARS epidemic, psychiatric problems related to the coronavirus disease 2019 pandemic may persist up to three years beyond the pandemic. The risk of long-term psychiatric symptoms and disorders was higher in healthcare workers and individuals who were quarantined.

Case Fatality[8]

Overall case fatality rate till date in India is around 2.5 to 3%. Presence of pneumonia appears to be the most important predictor of mortality. The most vulnerable population in which disease is likely to take a fatal course is that of the elderly, the diabetics, male gender, patients of chronic obstructive pulmonary disease, patients with heart disease, malignancy especially metastatic disease or haematologic or of lung, chronic kidney disease, obese subjects, hypertensives and any other chronic illness that can result in an immunocompromised state or compromised lung capacities. In a subset of 355 patients who died in Italy due to COVID-19, the mean number of pre-existing comorbidities was 2.7, and only 3 patients had no underlying condition.

Complications

- Acute respiratory distress syndrome (ARDS) is an important complication with severe disease and can manifest even in the beginning soon after the onset of dyspnoea. In a study of 138 patients mentioned above, ARDS was noted in 20% of the patients, at a median of 8 days after the symptom onset. Mechanical ventilation was required in 12.3%. In another study of 201 patients in Wuhan, 41% developed ARDS; age >65 years, diabetes mellitus, and hypertension were each associated with ARDS.[9]

- Other complications were arrhythmias, acute cardiac injury and shock in 17%, 7% and 9%, respectively, in one study. In a series of 21 severely ill patients admitted to the ICU in the United States, one-third developed cardiomyopathy.[9]

- Thromboembolic complications, including pulmonary embolism and acute stroke (even in patients younger than 50 years of age without risk factors), have also been reported.[9] Some patients with severe COVID-19 have laboratory evidence of an exuberant inflammatory response, similar to cytokine release syndrome, with persistent fevers, elevated inflammatory markers (e.g. D-dimer, ferritin), and elevated proinflammatory cytokines; these laboratory abnormalities have been associated with critical and fatal illnesses.

- Guillain-Barré syndrome has also been reported[9], with onset 5 to 10 days after initial symptoms.

- A multisystem inflammatory syndrome possibly associated with COVID-19, with clinical features similar to those of toxic shock syndrome and Kawasaki disease[5], has also been described in children.

Recovery

As per WHO, recovery time appears to be around two weeks for mild infections and three to six weeks for severe disease.[4]

REFERENCES

1. https://www.cdc.gov/coronavirus/2019-ncov/symptoms-testing/symptoms.html (as on 30th April 2020).
2. United States Centers for Disease Control and Prevention. Symptoms of Coronavirus. Available at: https//www.cdc.gov/coronavirus/2019-ncov/symptoms-testing/testing.html (as on April 28, 2020).
3. International Pulmonologists Consensus on COVID-19. Dr. Tinku Joseph, Dr. Mohammed Ashkan Moslehi, 2020.
4. https://www.who.int/health-topics/coronavirus#tab=tab_3 (as on 30th April 2020).
5. https://www.medscape.com/viewarticle/930180 (as on 18th May 2020).
6. Hao F, Tan W, Jiang L, et al. Do psychiatric patients experience more psychiatric symptoms during COVID-19 pandemic and lockdown? A Case-Control Study with Service and Research Implications for Immunopsychiatry. Brain Behav Immun. 2020 Apr 27. pii: S0889-1591(20)30626-7. doi: 10.1016/j.bbi.2020.04.069. [Epub ahead of print]
7. https://medicaldialogues.in/ent/news/loss-of-smell-and-taste-most-common-symptoms-in-covid-19-patients-with-high-recovery-rate-64827 (as on 10th May 2020)
8. Nikpouraghdam M, Jalali Farahani A, Alishiri G, et al. Epidemiological characteristics of coronavirus disease 2019 (COVID-19) patients in IRAN: A single center study. J Clin Virol 2020;127:104378. doi:10.1016/j.jcv.2020.104378
9. https://www.uptodate.com/contents/coronavirus-disease-2019-covid-19-epidemiology-virology-clinical-features-diagnosis-and-prevention?search=covid and source=search_result and selectedTitle=1~150 and usage_type=default and display_rank=1 (as on 10th may 2020).

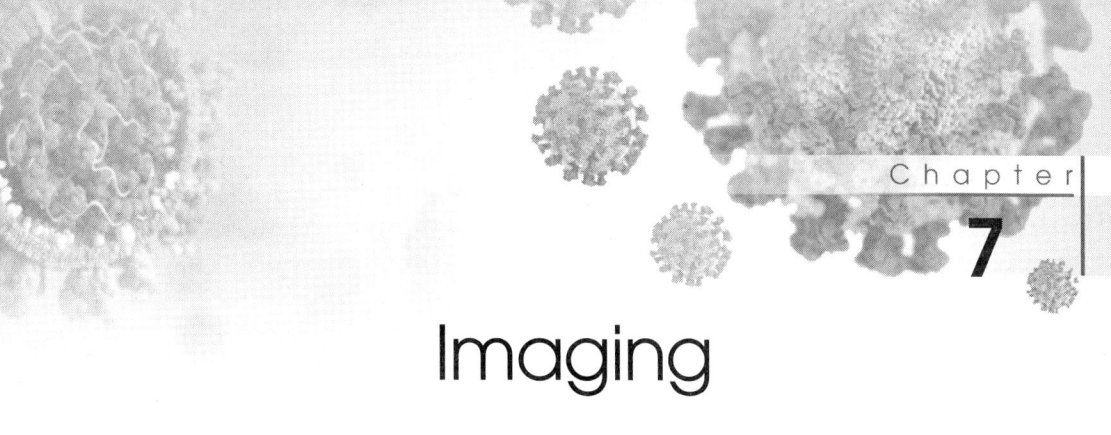

Imaging

Ishan Kumar, Adity Prakash, Ashish Verma

In December 2019, a novel coronavirus originated in the Wuhan city of Hubei province of China. The virus soon sprawled across multiple nations. The first case of coronavirus disease-19 (COVID-19) in India was reported on January 30, from Kerala. World Health Organization (WHO) declared the infection as a global pandemic and a public health emergency of international concern on 30 January 2020.[1]

The diagnosis of COVID-19 is mainly dependent on reverse transcriptase-polymerase chain reaction (RT-PCR) of respiratory samples, most commonly a nasal or an oropharyngeal swab. Many recent reports have suggested that RT-PCR may not always be positive leading to missing of a large number of cases. These cases may subsequently infect many greater numbers of people. This significantly downplays all the efforts being put into contain the spread.

ROLE OF RADIOLOGY: WHAT DATA TELLS US SO FAR

Most early studies from China encouraged the use of chest CT for screening patients with COVID-19. In fact, when China was at the peak of its epidemic, it officially broadened its definition of clinically diagnosed cases to include those cases with radiographic findings consistent with COVID-19. Thus, chest CT was used as a triage tool.[2]

Fang et al found sensitivity of chest CT to be much more than that of RT-PCR (98% vs 71%, respectively). The low efficiency of viral nucleic acid test could be due to low viral load in the patient, variations in testing kits from different manufacturers or due to incorrect collection, transportation or processing of samples. The study supported the use of chest CT for screening COVID-19 in patients with consistent clinical and epidemiological history, particularly when the RT-PCR tests are negative.[3] A study done on confirmed cases of COVID-19 comprising of passengers and crew members of "Diamond Princess" cruise ship showed that CT chest was positive in 54% of even asymptomatic cases.[4] A larger study by Ai T et al, comparing chest CT with RT-PCR, reaffirmed the high sensitivity of chest CT (97%) in picking up the lesions of the infection. However, they pointed out the pitfall of CT that was its low specificity (25%) because of overlap in its imaging findings with many other viral infections (H1N1).[5]

In fact, the radiological findings of COVID-19 are not a surprise for the radiologists as the findings are very similar to severe acute respiratory syndrome (SARS) virus of 2003 and Middle East respiratory syndrome (MERS) virus of 2012. The specificity of chest-CT for COVID-19 varies across different studies and the reported specificity ranges from 7 to 100%. One study found that the specificity improved to above 90% after proper training of the radiologist. Reports from USA have suggested that the sensitivity of chest CT could be between 80 and 90%. They have suggested sticking to RT-PCR owing to the low specificity of CT (60–70%) in COVID-19.[6] Kanne et al reported that up to 50% of patients with COVID-19 infection may have normal CT scans, especially on first two days after onset of symptoms, emphasizing the fact that a negative CT does not rule out the infection. However, they also acknowledged that the sensitivity of RT-PCR may be as low as 60–70%; therefore, patients with pneumonia due to COVID-19 may have lung abnormalities on chest CT but an initially negative RT-PCR.[7]

Chest CT may also have a role in prognostication of confirmed cases. A well-aerated lung on admission scan is associated with better prognosis independent of other clinical parameters. Those patients who show involvement of four or more lobes at baseline chest CT have more chance of an ICU admission and/or death.[8]

A meta-analysis comparing the diagnostic performance of chest CT and RT-PCR for COVID-19 found that CT had a low positive predictive value (1.5–30.7%) in countries with low prevalence of COVID-19. They highlighted that usage of chest CT in low prevalence regions could lead to large number of false positives and greater medical costs.[9]

Recommendations Regarding Role of Radiology

The **American College of Radiology (ACR)** states that the Centers for Disease Control (CDC) does not currently recommend chest X-ray (CXR) or CT to diagnose COVID-19 because of overlapping findings with other infections. Confirmation with a viral testing is required, even if the radiological findings are suggestive of COVID-19 on CXR or CT.[10]

The **British Society of Thoracic Imaging** also refutes any role for CT-imaging in COVID-19 unless the patient is seriously ill or PCR is unavailable. In confirmed cases of COVID-19, imaging (CXR and CT) may guide individual patient management decisions and deal with complications.[11]

The **Fleischner Society guidelines** state that imaging is indicated only in high-risk mild cases, moderate/severe cases and those who show worsening of respiratory status. Additionally, CT may be used in patients with functional impairment/hypoxaemia after recovery from COVID-19. Also, COVID-19 testing is indicated in patients incidentally found to have findings suggestive of COVID-19 on CT scan.[12]

The recommendations of **Indian Radiological and Imaging Association–Indian College of Radiology and Imaging (IRIA–ICRI)** sub-specialty group has focused mainly on portable radiographs and portable ultrasound. CT is not advocated generally as it is possible that the CT machine may become a spreader of infection. It is difficult to sterilize a CT machine (vs portable X-ray or a portable ultrasound machine). Most hospitals in India will not be able to provide a dedicated CT scanner for scanning exclusively COVID-19 patients. The transport of patients to CT room is an additional hurdle. As per the current **ICRI Chest Radiology Subspeciality group**, there is no imaging recommendation for either screening or for diagnosis of COVID-19. Imaging is also not recommended in mild cases except for those mild cases which have a high risk for developing severe disease (age >65 years, diabetes, cardiovascular disease, immunocompromised state, chronic liver/kidney/lung disease), if clinically needed.

The main role of imaging is for moderate/severe cases. CXR will provide a baseline status. CXR may be repeated based on clinical needs. However, a daily CXR is not needed. If the patient shows clinical/radiological deterioration, CXR and point of care ultrasound (POCUS) may be used to find the cause of worsening (ventilator-associated pneumonia (VAP), pulmonary thromboembolism, cardiac failure, etc.). CT is reserved only for those cases where CXR and POCUS are unable to explain the cause of worsening.[13,14]

Apart from its well-established roles in stratifying the severity of the infection, monitoring its progress and to look for complications, CT may find newer roles with further studies. As of now, most studies show the capacity of CT chest to emerge as a crucial tool for COVID-19. It helps in obtaining an initial probability of infection within seconds to minutes enabling immediate isolation of suspected cases. On the other hand, the RT-PCR test takes hours to days.

Also, it helps to address the problem of false negatives of RT-PCR. A patient with clinical features and imaging findings typical of COVID-19, but negative on RT-PCR test must still be kept in isolation till an alternative diagnosis is confirmed and a repeat RT-PCR may be considered. Amid the huge constraints on resources during the pandemic, there may be lack of testing kits. Some kits may be faulty. CT chest may help in such situations. Last but not the least, CT will have a definite role in monitoring response to various novel therapies being proposed for COVID-19. It will demonstrate whether and to what degree different treatment options impact the size, number and morphology of lung lesions. A suggested flowchart of COVID-19 suspects is presented in Fig. 7.1.

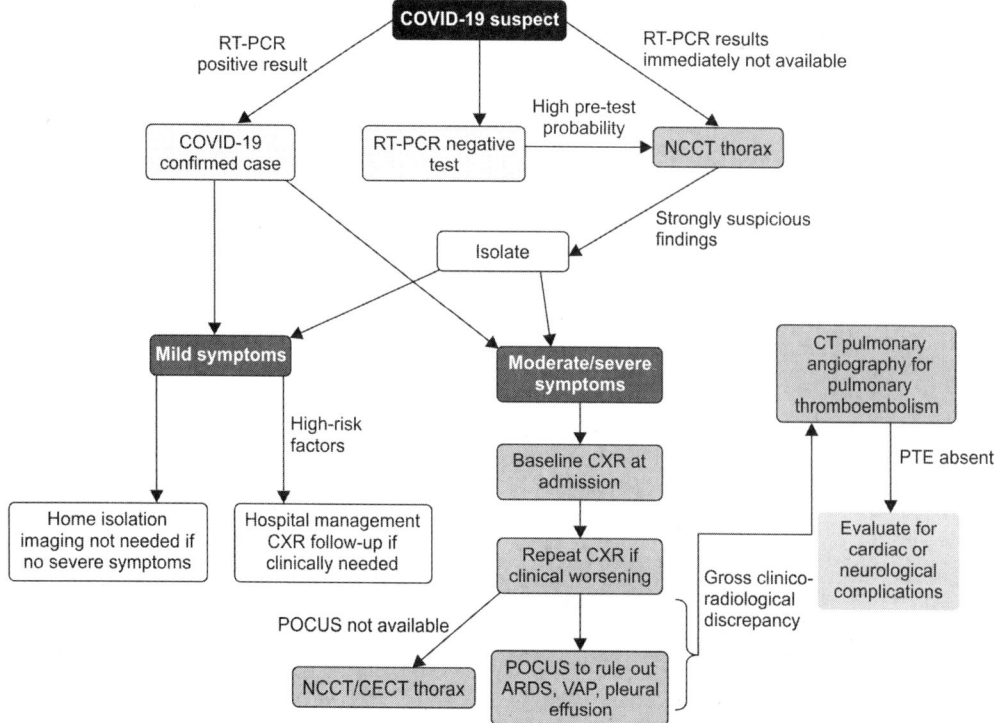

Fig. 7.1: Flowchart for management of suspected COVID-19

Radiological Findings

Chest X-ray

Although the sensitivity and specificity of chest X-ray in diagnosis of COVID-19 is modest, it may be the only imaging performed in these patients in majority of the cases. It can be performed in COVID-19 suspects as an initial triage tool, if there is a delay in laboratory confirmation or lack of testing facility in the vicinity to make a decision to place a patient in isolation. Presence of fever, shortness of breath, hypoxia (SpO_2 ≤94%) or increased respiratory rate ≥20/min are clinical features suspicious of COVID-19 in current situation. Moreover, chest X-ray performed in non-suspected patients can also reveal suspicion of COVID-19. Chest X-ray should be performed preferably using a portable digital radiographic (DR) equipment. As much as possible, 6 feet distance from the patients should be kept.

Some recommend positioning the X-ray tube outside the open door of the cubicle, while the medical staff with PPE positions the patient upright and places the cassette/detector. Studies recommend all the chest radiographs performed during the pandemic to be reported using CX-Reporting system.[15,16]

1. CX-NP—no features of pneumonia.
2. CX-IP — indeterminate features of pneumonia (findings suggestive of fibrotic disease or pulmonary oedema)
3. CX-FP—focal pneumonia (less likely to be COVID-19)
4. CX-MP—bilateral and multifocal pneumonia (most characteristic of COVID-19)

Features such as lobar/sublobar consolidations, nodules, pneumothorax are more likely to suggest other diagnosis.

CT Scan

As per current recommendations, CT should not be used for screening or diagnosis of COVID suspected patients and should be reserved only for RT-PCR negative case with a clinical history strongly suspicious of COVID (contact with COVID-19 positive case or having clinical deterioration). Also, CT should not be done routinely for a proven COVID-19 cases and should be reserved to confirm a specific clinical diagnosis such as ARDS, pulmonary embolism or CT head for acute necrotizing encephalopathy.

The most common radiological findings that have been reported are bilateral (76%) ground-glass opacities (GGO) (86%) in a peripheral distribution (33%). Other findings include peripheral consolidations, crazy paving pattern, reverse halo pattern, subpleural curvilinear opacities and rounded opacities[17] (Fig. 7.2).

Findings such as pleural thickening, pleural effusion, discrete nodules, tree-in-bud, cavitations and lymphadenopathy have been described as consistently absent in all cases except one case in which Kong et al. described a small solitary cavitation in one of the follow-up scan of a positive case.[18] Follow-up imaging series of patients show that ground-glass opacities are the predominant finding early in the course of the disease. The radiological findings are at their peak at about 9–11 days after onset of symptoms. As the disease progresses, ground-glass opacities change into consolidations and thus, consolidations become the predominant lesion. Most of the patients will show resolution of imaging findings after a month or beyond. However, a fraction of

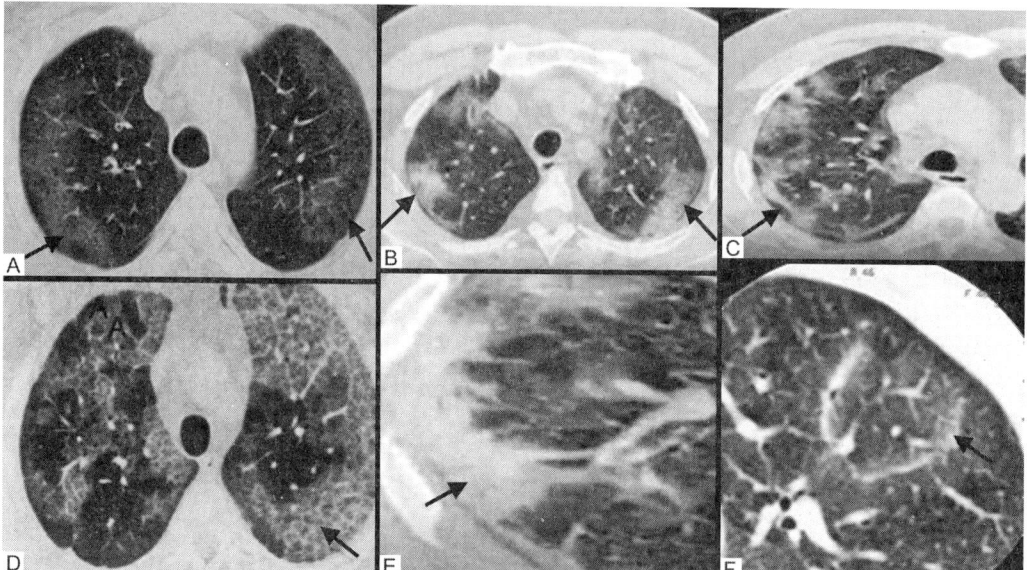

Fig. 7.2: Common CT findings associated with COVID-19: (A) Bilateral ground-glass opacities; (B) Bilateral peripheral consolidations; (C) Linear subpleural opacities; (D) Crazy paving pattern; (E) Subpleural consolidations; (F) Reverse halo "atoll" sign.

patients will progress to diffuse alveolar damage, manifested radiologically as diffuse infiltrates of acute respiratory distress syndrome (ARDS).[7] Pulmonary thrombo-embolism also has been reported to be associated with COVID-19 and requires CT pulmonary angiography for confirmation.

The British Society of Thoracic Imaging (BSTI) has enlisted four patterns of imaging appearances based on the confidence of a diagnosis consistent with COVID-19.

1. A **classic** pattern (100% confidence for COVID-19) shows a lower lobe predominant, peripheral predominant, multiple, bilateral foci of GGO with or without crazy paving, peripheral consolidation, air bronchograms or a reverse halo.
2. A **probable** pattern (71–99% confidence for COVID-19) has peripheral and bronchocentric consolidations but GGOs are scarce.
3. An **indeterminate** pattern (<70% confidence for COVID-19) does not in any category or may manifest above patterns but the clinical context is wrong.
4. A **non-COVID** pattern (70% confidence for alternative) is a pattern that is inconsistent with COVID-19 and includes findings such as lobar pneumonia, cavitation, tree-in-bud, lymphadenopathy, effusions, established pulmonary fibrosis (Fig. 7.3).

A CT severity index may be given as a part of report to classify the disease as either mild or moderate/severe:

- **Mild** disease: Up to 3 focal abnormalities, 3 cm in maximum diameter
- **Moderate/severe** disease: More than 3 focal abnormalities or maximum diameter more than 3 cm.[11]

A recommendation by Indian Radiological and Imaging Association proposes a visual assessment of overall area of lung and categorization as <25% (score 1), 25–50% (score 2), 50–75% (score 3) and >75% (score 4).[19]

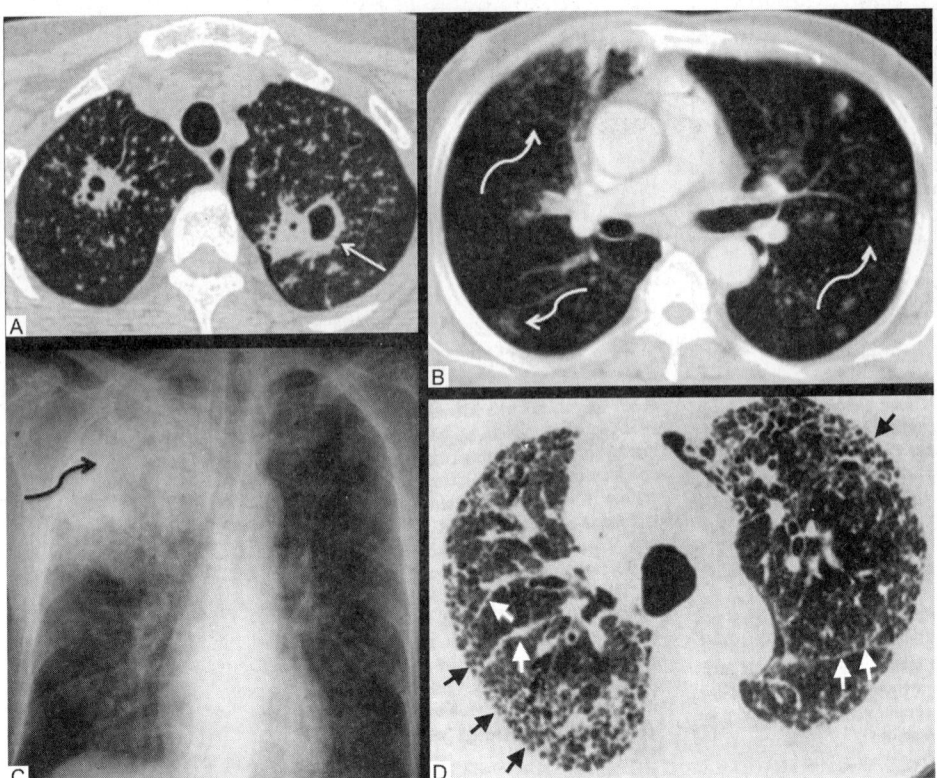

Fig. 7.3: Radiological features not present in COVID suggesting alternative diagnosis: (A) Cavitary lesions; (B) Tree in bud nodules; (C) Lobar consolidation; (D) Fibrotic lung with honeycombing

Point of Care Ultrasound

Role of sonography in the current pandemic is evolving, especially in monitoring the patients in ICU. It is re-emphasized that USG is not a diagnostic or a screening tool for COVID-19. Sonography should be performed using convex or linear probe with 8 intercoastal scans placing the transducer in upper and lower mid-clavicular and mid-axillary lines bilaterally.[20] Posterior chest may be difficult to scan in supine patients and not covered in minimum recommendation but should be included, if the patient can attain an upright position.

USG findings described in COVID-19 patients are B-lines (comet tail) artifacts, interrupted pleural line, subpleural consolidation, sonographic air bronchograms, pleural effusion and reduced Doppler flow (Fig. 7.4).[21]

A sonographic severity scoring has been proposed:[20]
- Score 0: Continuous pleural line with normal horizontal A-line artifacts.
- Score 1: Indented and mildly irregular pleural line and presence of B-lines.
- Score 2: Interrupted pleural lines with subpleural consolidations.
- Score 3: Coalescent B-lines, white lung with or without large consolidations.

ESTABLISHING A SAFE WORKFLOW

Regardless of the indication, strict infection control protocol must be adhered to while imaging all such cases. The confirmed COVID case must be scanned at last, at the end

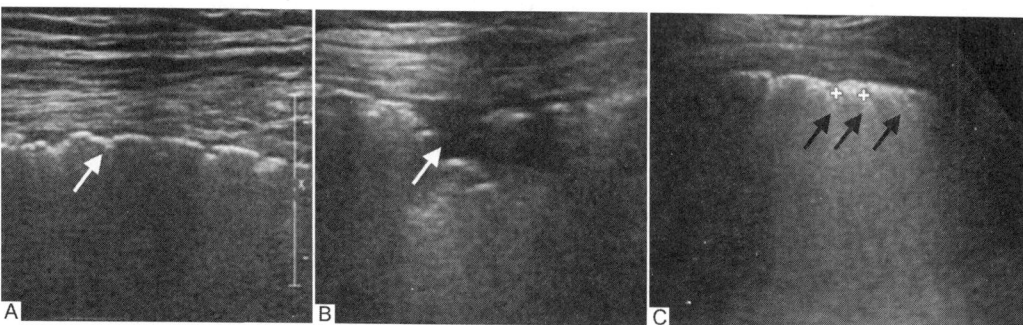

Fig. 7.4: Ultrasonographic findings expected in COVID-19 patients: (A) Interrupted and indented pleural line; (B) Subpleural consolidation; (C) B-lines artifacts

of the day. The patient should be wearing an N95 mask. The patient should enter the scanner area through a separate door. The doctor and technicians must wear the complete personal protective equipment including double gloves, N95 mask, gown, shoe covers, goggles, hood. One operator can help in proper positioning of the patient while another technician sits at the console. A glass wall should be used to give instructions to the patient. The machine and the entire room should be sterilized after each case and the CT room should be closed for one hour after the scan to allow passive ventilation.[14] A trivial error in the infection control protocol may come with a heavy price.

Chest X-ray and ultrasound should be performed only using bedside portable X-ray and sonographic equipment. Ultrasound transducers should be first cleaned using tap water, non-abrasive detergent and wiping the transducer cable with LLD wipes. After drying the transducer with towel, disinfection should be done using 2.4–3.2% glutaraldehyde products (Cidex) or sodium hypochlorite 0.21% (Antisapril Blu 2%) or ethanol 80–95%.[22]

The COVID isolation ward should ideally have a dedicated portable X-ray equipment. Radiographs of the suspected patients should be first performed followed by confirmed patients. The portable machine and the cassette/detector should be wiped with alcohol rub and the cassette/detector should be covered with two layers of plastic. X-ray should be performed after donning PPE. If cassettes need to be taken back to the department, sanitization with isopropyl alcohol should be ensured.

Extrapulmonary Manifestations

Cardiac involvement: Accumulated evidence suggests that cardiac involvement is common, particularly in a patient hospitalized with COVID-19 disease although there is scarcity of a systematic study to investigate the same. In a case report of a COVID-19 with cardiac involvement, cardiac magnetic resonance imaging (MRI) patient demonstrated increased wall thickness with diffuse biventricular hypokinesis, especially in the apical segments, severe LV dysfunction (LVEF of 35%) and diffuse oedema, and the slow gadolinium washout are consistent with acute myopericarditis.[23]

Brain involvement: Although there is clinical evidence of olfactory dysfunction in many patients, MRI of the olfactory bulbs were within normal limits in those patients. A case report shows acute haemorrhagic necrotizing encephalopathy characterized by haemorrhagic rim enhancing lesions within the bilateral thalami, medial temporal lobes, and subinsular regions.[24]

CONCLUSION

This review attempts to familiarize the radiologists and clinicians to the radiological appearance and recommendations to optimize the use of radiological facilities in the management of COVID-19 patients. COVID-19 is not the first pandemic affecting the mankind and, in all probability, it will not be the last. There are important lessons to be taken from this disease, the foremost being expansion of the radiological infrastructure of all the hospitals. All the hospitals should invest in communicable disease ICU and quarantine wards with dedicated bedside USG, X-ray facilities and if possible portable CT units.

Acknowledgement: The authors thank Dr Manoj Ranjan, consultant radiologist, Heritage Hospital, Varanasi, for providing the image of a suspected COVID-19 patient.

REFERENCES

1. World Health Organization. Coronavirus disease (COVID-19) outbreak. https:// www.who.int/westernpacific/emergencies/covid-19. Accessed April 18, 2020

2. National Health Commission of the People's Republic of China website. Diagnosis and treatment of novel coronavirus infection (trial version 6). Published February 18, 2020.

3. Fang Y, Zhang H, et al. Sensitivity of chest CT for COVID-19: Comparison to RT-PCR. Radiology 2020. Doi: 10.1148/radiol.2020200432

4. Inui S, Fujikawa A, Jitsu M, Kunishima N, Watanabe S, Suzuki Y et al. Chest CT findings in cases from the cruise ship "Diamond Princess" with coronavirus disease 2019 (COVID-19). Radiology: Cardiothoracic Imaging 2020;2(2):e200110.

5. Ai T, Yang Z, Hou H, et al. Correlation of chest CT and RT-PCR testing in coronavirus disease 2019 (COVID-19) in China: A report of 1014 cases. Radiology 2020;200642.

6. Mossa-Basha M, Meltzer C, Kim D, Tuite M, Kolli K, Tan B. Radiology department preparedness for COVID-19: Radiology Scientific expert panel. Radiology 2020;200988.

7. Kanne J. Chest CT Findings in 2019 Novel Coronavirus (2019-nCoV) Infections from Wuhan, China: Key Points for the Radiologist. Radiology. 2020;295(1):16–17.

8. Colombi D, Bodini F, Petrini M, Maffi G, Morelli N, Milanese G et al. Well-aerated lung on admitting chest CT to predict adverse outcome in COVID-19 pneumonia. Radiology 2020;201433.

9. Kim H, Hong H, Yoon S. Diagnostic performance of CT and reverse transcriptase-polymerase chain reaction for coronavirus disease 2019: A meta-analysis. Radiology 2020;201343.

10. ACR recommendations for the use of chest radiography and computed tomography (CT) for suspected COVID-19 infection [Internet]. Acr Org 2020 [cited 7 April 2020].

11. Bsti.org.uk. 2020 Available from: https://www.bsti.org.uk/media/resources/files/ BSTI_COVID-19_Radiology_Guidance_v1_13.03.20_9kzNSRs.pdf

12. Rubin G, Ryerson C, Haramati L, et al. The role of chest imaging in patient management during the COVID-19 pandemic: A multinational consensus statement from the Fleischner Society. Chest 2020.

13. Mohfw.gov.in.2020. https://www.mohfw.gov.in/pdf/Guidelineson Clinical Management of COVID-19 12020.p

14. Imaging in COVID-19 patients: Indian guidelines recommendations of Indian Radiological and Imaging Association.

15. Reporting format available on. covid19action-radiology.github.io

16. Yoon et al. Chest radiographic and CT findings of the 2019 novel coronavirus disease (COVID-19): Analysis of nine patients treated in Korea. Korean J Radiol 2020;21(4):494–500.

17. Chung M, Bernheim A, Mei X, Zhang N, Huang M, Zeng X, et al. CT imaging features of 2019 novel coronavirus (2019-nCoV). Radiology 2020;295(1):202–07.

18. Kong W, Agarwal P. Chest imaging appearance of COVID-19 infection. Radiology: Cardiothoracic Imaging 2020;2(1):e200028.

19. Naranje P, Bhalla AS. Proposal for severity grading of COVID-19. Endorsed by Indian Radiological and Imaging Association.

20. Soldati G, Smargiassi A, et al. Proposal for international standardization of the use of lung ultrasound for COVID-19 patients; a simple, quantitative, reproducible method. J Ultrasound Med 2020. doi:10.1002/jum.15285.

21. Huang Yi, Wang, Sihan, Liu, et al. A preliminary study on the ultrasonic manifestations of peripulmonary lesions of non-critical novel coronavirus pneumonia (COVID-19) (Feb 26, 2020). Available at SRN: https://ssrn.com/abstract=3544750

22. Poon LC, et al. ISUOG Safety Committee Position Statement: Safe performance of obstetric and gynecological scans and equipment cleaning in the context of COVID-19. March 2020.

23. Nciardi RM, Lupi L, Zaccone G, et al. Cardiac Involvement in a Patient With Coronavirus Disease 2019 (COVID-19) [published online ahead of print, 2020 Mar 27]. JAMA Cardiol 2020;10.1001/jamacardio.2020.1096. doi:10.1001/jamacardio.2020.1096

24. Poyiadji N, Shahin G, Noujaim D, Stone M, Patel S, Griffith B. COVID-19-associated Acute Hemorrhagic Necrotizing Encephalopathy: CT and MRI Features [published online ahead of print, 2020 Mar 31]. Radiology 2020;201187. doi:10.1148/radiol.2020201187.

Management of COVID-19

Akhilesh Tiwari, Deepak Kumar Shah

COVID-19 may present with mild, moderate, or severe illness; the latter includes severe pneumonia, ARDS, sepsis and septic shock. Early identification of those with severe manifestations allows for immediate optimized supportive care treatments and safe, rapid admission (or referral) to intensive care unit according to national protocols.

DEFINITIONS OF PATIENTS WITH COVID-19

1. **Severe acute respiratory infections (SARI):** An ARI with history of fever or measured temperature ≥38°C and cough; onset within the last ~10 days and requiring hospitalization.

2. **Uncomplicated illness:** These patients have non-specific symptoms such as fever, cough, sore throat, nasal congestion, malaise, headache. The elderly and immunosuppressed may present with atypical symptoms. These patients do not have any signs of dehydration, sepsis or shortness of breath.

3. **Mild pneumonia:** Patient with pneumonia and no signs of severe pneumonia. Child with non-severe pneumonia has cough or difficulty in breathing or fast breathing (fast breathing rate means: <2 months—≥60 breaths/min; 2–11 months—≥50 breaths/min; 1–5 years—≥40 breaths/min and no signs of severe pneumonia).

4. **Severe pneumonia—*adolescent or adult*:** Fever or suspected respiratory infection, plus one of the following: Respiratory rate >30 breaths/min, severe respiratory distress, SpO_2 <90% on room air. ***Child*** with cough or difficulty in breathing, plus at least one of the following: Central cyanosis or SpO_2 <90%; severe respiratory distress (e.g. grunting, chest indrawing); signs of pneumonia with any of the following danger signs: Inability to breastfeed or drink, lethargy or unconsciousness, or convulsions. Other signs of pneumonia may be present: Chest indrawing, fast breathing. The diagnosis is mainly clinical, chest imaging can exclude complications.

5. **Acute respiratory distress syndrome:** New or worsening respiratory symptoms within one week of known clinical insult. Respiratory failure not fully explained by cardiac failure or fluid overload. Need objective assessment (e.g. echocardiography) to exclude hydrostatic cause of oedema, if no risk factor present. Chest imaging shows bilateral opacities, not fully explained by effusions, lobar or lung collapse, or nodules.

– *Mild ARDS:* 200 mmHg $<paO_2/FiO_2 \leq 300$ mmHg (with PEEP or CPAP ≥ 5 cm H_2O, or non-ventilated).

– *Moderate ARDS:* 100 mmHg $<paO_2/FiO_2 \leq 200$ mmHg with PEEP ≥ 5 cm H_2O, or non-ventilated).

– *Severe ARDS*: $PaO_2/FiO_2 \leq 100$ mmHg with PEEP ≥ 5 cm H_2O, or non-ventilated.

6. **Sepsis—*adults*:** Life-threatening organ dysfunction caused by a dysregulated host response to suspected or proven infection, with organ dysfunction. Signs of organ dysfunction include: Altered mental status, difficult or fast breathing, low oxygen saturation, reduced urine output, fast heart rate, weak pulse, cold extremities or low blood pressure, skin mottling, or laboratory evidence of coagulopathy, thrombocytopenia, acidosis, high lactate or hyperbilirubinaemia.

Children: Suspected or proven infection and ≥ 2 SIRS criteria, of which one must be abnormal temperature or white blood cell count.

7. **Septic shock—*adults*:** Persisting hypotension despite volume resuscitation, requiring vasopressors to maintain MAP ≥ 65 mmHg and serum lactate level <2 mmol/l.

Children: Any hypotension (SBP <5th centile or >2 SD below normal for age) or 2–3 of the following: Altered mental state; bradycardia or tachycardia (HR <90 bpm or >160 bpm in infants and HR <70 bpm or >150 bpm in children); prolonged capillary refill (>2 sec) or warm vasodilation with bounding pulses; tachypnoea; mottled skin or petechial or purpuric rash; increased lactate; oliguria; hyperthermia or hypothermia.

8. **Close contact:**
   a. Healthcare-associated exposure, including providing direct care for COVID-19 patients, working with healthcare workers infected with COVID-19, visiting patients or staying in the same close environment of a COVID-19 patient.
   b. Working together in close proximity or sharing the same classroom environment with a COVID-19 patient.
   c. Travelling together with COVID-19 patient in any kind of conveyance.
   d. Living in the same household with a COVID-19 patient.[1]

COVID-19 PNEUMONITIS

Broadly, COVID-19 pneumonitis can be divided into two primary phenotypes: L-type and H-type.

COVID-19 Pneumonia—Type L

At the beginning, COVID-19 pneumonia presents with the following characteristics.

- **Low elastance**: Nearly normal compliance.
- **Low ventilation-to-perfusion (VA/Q) ratio**: Hypoxaemia may be best explained by the loss of regulation of perfusion and by loss of hypoxic vasoconstriction.
- **Low lung weight.** Only ground-glass densities are present on CT scan, primarily located subpleurally and along the lung fissures.
- **Low lung recruitability**. The amount of non-aerated tissue is very low.

COVID-19 Pneumonia—Type H (typical ARDS-like picture)

- High elastance
- High right-to-left shunt
- High lung weight

Note: It is to be noted that these are not mutually exclusive but may represent the same disease process in different stages of evolution.

The combination of a negative inspiratory intrathoracic pressure and increased lung permeability due to inflammation results in interstitial lung oedema (leading cause of patient **self-inflicted lung injury (P-SILI)** and is responsible for transition from L-type to H-type.

The typical imaging features are found in L phenotype.

CLINICAL MANAGEMENT[2]

Indications for Admission

COVID Care Centres

Confirmed cases with mild disease.

Hospital Admission

COVID ward: The following criteria may be applied to consider for admission (any one of the following):

1. Respiratory rate >24/min
2. SpO_2 <94% on room air
3. Those at high risk for severe disease:
   a. Age >60 years
   b. Cardiovascular disease including hypertension
   c. Diabetes mellitus/other immunocompromised states
   d. Chronic lung/liver/kidney disease
   e. Cerebrovascular disease

COVID ICU: The following criteria may be applied to consider for admission (any one of the following):

1. Moderate/severe ARDS
2. Multiorgan dysfunction
3. Shock
4. Transfer from ward to ICU, if needs mechanical ventilation/closer monitoring.

However, the final decision to admit and triage is at the discretion of the treating physician.

Management of Mild Cases

Mild cases are those with low grade fever/cough/malaise/rhinorrhoea/sore throat without any shortness of breath.

a. Admission in COVID care centres
b. Contact and droplet precautions, strict hand hygiene

c. Symptomatic treatment

d. Tab hydroxychloroquine 400 mg BD for 1 day followed by 400 mg OD for 4 days in patients with high-risk factors for severe disease may be considered.

e. Antibiotics and antivirals as per clinician's discretion (to cover community acquired pneumonia including atypical pneumonia and influenza)

f. Low threshold for transfer of patients with high-risk factor for severe disease to designated hospitals.

Management of Hospitalized Cases in Ward

General Measures

a. Symptomatic treatment

b. Antibiotics and antivirals as per clinician's discretion (to cover community acquired pneumonia including atypical pneumonia and influenza)

c. Maintain euvolemia

d. Tab hydroxychloroquine 400 mg BD for 1 day followed by 400 mg OD for 4 days in patients with high-risk factors for severe disease may be considered.

Clinical Monitoring

a. Work of breathing

b. Excessive inspiratory efforts (requiring accessory muscles of respiration, large volume tidal breaths, air hunger)

c. Oxygen requirement

d. Vital signs

Laboratory Evaluation[3,8]

Routine: CBC with differentials, LFT, KFT, coagulation profile, urine R/M

Predictive and prognostic markers: CRP, LDH, ferritin, D-dimer, Troponin I

Abnormality	Possible threshold
Elevations in:	
• D-dimer	>1000 ng/ml (normal range: <500 ng/ml)
• CRP	>100 mg/l (normal range: <8.0 mg/l)
• LDH	>245 units/l (normal range: 110 to 210 units/l)
• Troponin	>2 × the upper limit of normal (normal range for troponin T high sensitivity: Females 0 to 9 ng/l; males 0 to 14 ng/l)
• Ferritin	>500 µg/l (normal range: Females 10 to 200 µg/l; males 30 to 300 µg/l)
• CPK	>2 × the upper limit of normal (normal range: 40 to 150 units/l)
Decrease in:	
• Absolute lympho-cyte count	<800/µl (normal range for age >21 years: 1800 to 7700 µl)

Oxygen Therapy in COVID-19 Pneumonitis

Non-Ventilatory Management (in patients with hypoxaemia and low work of breathing)

- Target SpO_2 92–96% (88–92% in patients with COPD).
- Preferable devices for delivering oxygen: Non-rebreathing face mask, venturi-mask and high flow nasal cannula (HFNC) (if available).
- Assessment of severity of hypoxemia/shunt: If patient achieves an SpO_2 >95% at 15 l/min O_2 the shunt fraction is mild. Failure to achieve this indicates a moderate–severe shunt fraction.
- If the target is not achieved/maintained with the above-mentioned devices, cautious trials of CPAP via oronasal mask/NIV via helmet interface may be given.
- Try to achieve targets with lowest possible PEEP.
- Use of CPAP/NIV requires intensive monitoring for any increase in work of breathing/large tidal volume breaths [to prevent self-inflicted lung injury (SILI)] and haemodynamic instability.

  Note:
  - NIV is associated with high failure rates, particularly in *de novo* respiratory failure.
  - NIV without helmet interface is associated with greater risks of aerosolization leading to higher exposure of healthcare workers.
  - Placing a surgical mask over nasal cannula (NC) may help in reducing dispersion.

Anticoagulation

- All hospitalized patients should be started on prophylactic LMWH (e.g. enoxaparin 1 mg/kg per day subcutaneously), if not contraindicated, and no high-risk factors for bleeding are present.
- Bleeding risk should be estimated with well-validated risk scores (e.g. HAS-BLED score of ≤3 signifies a higher bleeding risk).
- In patients who are admitted to ICU, consideration should be given to therapeutic dose LMWH (e.g. enoxaparin 1 mg/kg SC BD), if not at high risk of bleeding.

Specific Therapy

No specific antivirals have been definitively proven to be effective as per currently available data. Drugs which have been tried in clinical trial settings include:

a. Hydroxychloroquine/chloroquine

b. Lopinavir/ritonavir

c. Remdesivir

d. Nitazoxanide

e. Ivermectin

Note:

a. Remdesivir, a drug originally developed to treat Ebola viruses showed promising *in vitro* results. It is now FDA approved drug (1 May 2020) for the treatment of suspected or confirmed COVID-19 in adults and children hospitalized with severe disease.

b. (b) Convalescent plasma therapy (not approved by ICMR till now).

c. (c) **IL-6 pathway inhibitors:** Tocilizumab is an interleukin (IL)-6 receptor inhibitor. Elevated IL-6 levels have been described in patients with severe COVID-19, and case reports have described good outcomes with tocilizumab.

Vaccines

- The primary target in developing coronavirus vaccines has been the spike protein (S protein), *in vivo*, most important antigen for triggering an immune response.
- Use of Bacillus Calmette-Guérin (BCG) immunization for prevention of COVID-19 is undergoing clinical trials.
- The trial began in Oxford, with the first two of 800 healthy volunteers recruited for the study being injected with a new vaccine, **ChAdOx1 nCoV-19.**[9]

Role of Steroids

Steroids may be considered in a defined subgroup of patients including:

a. Patients with critical disease (admitted in the ICU)

b. Given the potential for delayed viral clearance, the duration of steroid use should be limited to 3 to 5 days (with no tapering) in low to moderate doses (1–2 mg/kg/day).

Supportive Treatment in Critically Ill Patients

a. Head end elevation (30 to 45°)

b. Oral hygiene with mouthwash

c. Glycaemic control to maintain blood sugar between 140 and 180 mg/dl.

d. Ulcer prophylaxis with proton pump inhibitors

e. LMWH for thromboprophylaxis

f. Foley's catheter and Ryle's tube placement

g. Central venous catheter (CVC) insertion

h. Pressure ulcer prevention by position change every 2 hourly

FLOWCHART OF CLINICAL GUIDANCE FOR MANAGEMENT OF COVID-19[2]

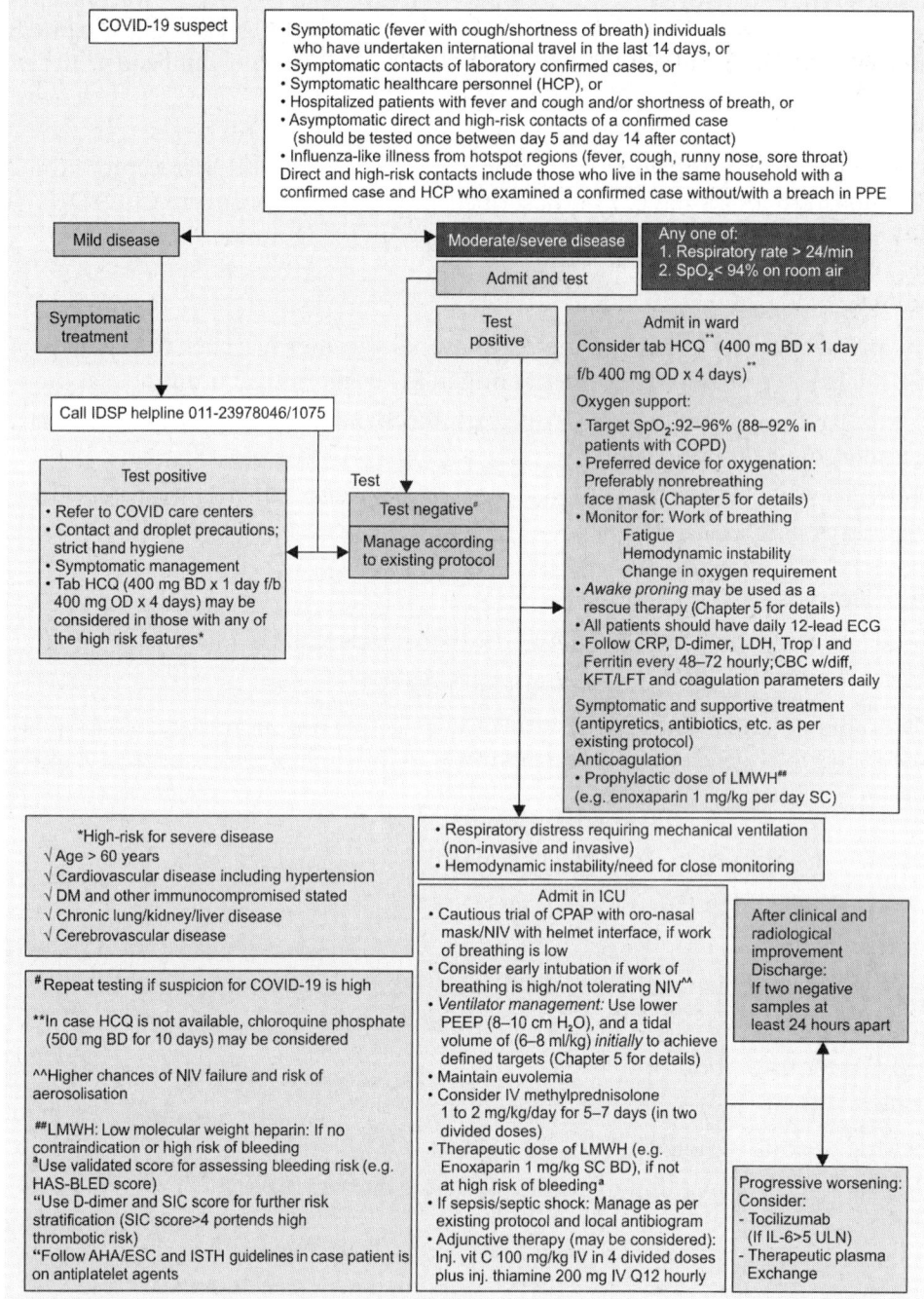

COVID-19 suspect
- Symptomatic (fever with cough/shortness of breath) individuals who have undertaken international travel in the last 14 days, or
- Symptomatic contacts of laboratory confirmed cases, or
- Symptomatic healthcare personnel (HCP), or
- Hospitalized patients with fever and cough and/or shortness of breath, or
- Asymptomatic direct and high-risk contacts of a confirmed case (should be tested once between day 5 and day 14 after contact)
- Influenza-like illness from hotspot regions (fever, cough, runny nose, sore throat)
Direct and high-risk contacts include those who live in the same household with a confirmed case and HCP who examined a confirmed case without/with a breach in PPE

Mild disease

Moderate/severe disease

Any one of:
1. Respiratory rate > 24/min
2. SpO_2 < 94% on room air

Admit and test

Symptomatic treatment

Test positive

Admit in ward
Consider tab HCQ** (400 mg BD x 1 day f/b 400 mg OD x 4 days)**

Oxygen support:
- Target SpO_2:92–96% (88–92% in patients with COPD)
- Preferred device for oxygenation: Preferably nonrebreathing face mask (Chapter 5 for details)
- Monitor for: Work of breathing
   Fatigue
   Hemodynamic instability
   Change in oxygen requirement
- *Awake proning* may be used as a rescue therapy (Chapter 5 for details)
- All patients should have daily 12-lead ECG
- Follow CRP, D-dimer, LDH, Trop I and Ferritin every 48–72 hourly;CBC w/diff, KFT/LFT and coagulation parameters daily

Symptomatic and supportive treatment (antipyretics, antibiotics, etc. as per existing protocol)
Anticoagulation
- Prophylactic dose of LMWH## (e.g. enoxaparin 1 mg/kg per day SC)

Call IDSP helpline 011-23978046/1075

Test positive
- Refer to COVID care centers
- Contact and droplet precautions; strict hand hygiene
- Symptomatic management
- Tab HCQ (400 mg BD x 1 day f/b 400 mg OD x 4 days) may be considered in those with any of the high risk features*

Test

Test negative*

Manage according to existing protocol

***High-risk for severe disease**
√ Age > 60 years
√ Cardiovascular disease including hypertension
√ DM and other immunocompromised stated
√ Chronic lung/kidney/liver disease
√ Cerebrovascular disease

Repeat testing if suspicion for COVID-19 is high

**In case HCQ is not available, chloroquine phosphate (500 mg BD for 10 days) may be considered

^^Higher chances of NIV failure and risk of aerosolisation

##LMWH: Low molecular weight heparin: If no contraindication or high risk of bleeding
ªUse validated score for assessing bleeding risk (e.g. HAS-BLED score)
ᵇUse D-dimer and SIC score for further risk stratification (SIC score>4 portends high thrombotic risk)
ᶜFollow AHA/ESC and ISTH guidelines in case patient is on antiplatelet agents

- Respiratory distress requiring mechanical ventilation (non-invasive and invasive)
- Hemodynamic instability/need for close monitoring

Admit in ICU
- Cautious trial of CPAP with oro-nasal mask/NIV with helmet interface, if work of breathing is low
- Consider early intubation if work of breathing is high/not tolerating NIV^^
- *Ventilator management:* Use lower PEEP (8–10 cm H_2O), and a tidal volume of (6–8 ml/kg) *initially* to achieve defined targets (Chapter 5 for details)
- Maintain euvolemia
- Consider IV methylprednisolone 1 to 2 mg/kg/day for 5–7 days (in two divided doses)
- Therapeutic dose of LMWH (e.g. Enoxaparin 1 mg/kg SC BD), if not at high risk of bleedingª
- If sepsis/septic shock: Manage as per existing protocol and local antibiogram
- Adjunctive therapy (may be considered): Inj. vit C 100 mg/kg IV in 4 divided doses plus inj. thiamine 200 mg IV Q12 hourly

After clinical and radiological improvement Discharge:
If two negative samples at least 24 hours apart

Progressive worsening:
Consider:
- Tocilizumab (If IL-6>5 ULN)
- Therapeutic plasma Exchange

NOTE

Category C Drugs

1. Chloroquine – azithromycin/levofloxacin: QT prolongation/hypoglycaemia
2. Chloroquine – aspirin/linezolid: QT prolongation/hypoglycaemia

X: Avoid combination, D: Consider treatment modification, C: Monitor therapy

REFERENCES

1. www.mohfw.gov.in Revised Guidelines on Clinical Management of COVID-19.
2. www.aiims.edu Information Related to COVID-19–AIIMS.
3. Guan WY, Ni ZY, Hu Y, et al. Clinical characteristics of coronavirus disease 2019 in China. N Engl J Med 2020.
4. Huang C, Wang Y, Li X, et al. Clinical features of patients infected with 2019 novel coronavirus in Wuhan, China. Lancet 2020; 395:497.
5. Zhou F, Yu T, Du R, et al. Clinical course and risk factors for mortality of adult inpatients with COVID-19 in Wuhan, China: a retrospective cohort study. Lancet 2020; 395:1054.
6. Wang D, Hu B, Hu C, et al. Clinical characteristics of 138 hospitalized patients with 2019 novel coronavirus-infected pneumonia in Wuhan, China. JAMA 2020.
7. Wu Z, McGoogan JM. Characteristics of and important lessons from the coronavirus disease 2019 (COVID-19) outbreak in China: Summary of a report of 72,314 cases from the Chinese Center for Disease Control and Prevention. JAMA 2020.
8. Ruan Q, Yang K, Wang W, et al. Clinical predictors of mortality due to COVID-19 based on an analysis of data of 150 patients from Wuhan, China. Intensive Care Med 2020.
9. http://research.ox.ac.uk/

Critical Care and Ventilator Support

Rajeev Kumar Dubey, Akhilesh Tiwari, Pallavi Gupta

Coronavirus disease 19 (COVID-19) has become a global pandemic. Usually the disease takes a mild and self-limiting course in approximately 81% of cases. It is estimated that around 14% of patients become severely ill and around 5% of the patients develop critical or life-threatening illness; it is, therefore, the patients belonging to these two classes combined will require intensive care unit (ICU) admission.[1] The progress of the disease is usually so rapid that there is no distinct demarcation between the severe illness and critical illness. The patients who develop severe illness and need admission into an intensive care unit are usually elderly (>60 years old) with one or more comorbidities such as hypertension, any other cardiovascular disease, diabetes mellitus or hepatic or renal dysfunction.[2,3] After around 7 to 10 days of the onset of disease, the usual clinical manifestations of fever, headache, dry cough, pneumonia can rapidly progress to acute respiratory distress syndrome (ARDS), myocardial dysfunction, dysrhythmias, septic shock, refractory metabolic acidosis, acute renal failure and coagulopathy.[4,5]

There is an imperative need to strengthen an integrated training to attain homogeneity of clinical cognition, optimization of critical care resource allocation and delivery of intensive care services. Standardized operating procedures (SOPs) need to be developed. A multidisciplinary team approach is essential that should comprise experts from intensive care, respiratory medicine, nephrology, endocrinology, pathology and infectious diseases. It is also worthwhile to implement infection prevention and control (IPC) measures so as to prevent further transmission and safeguard the healthcare workers, especially when no definitive treatment or post-exposure prophylaxis is available. Therefore, regular staff education and training are the most effective modalities to improve ICU preparedness.

BASIC INFECTION PREVENTION AND CONTROL (IPC) PRINCIPLES IN ICU

Coronaviruses are enveloped viruses with a single positive-stranded RNA genome and their main transmission route is via droplets and close contact. While novel coronavirus (nCoV) appears to be predominantly spread by large respiratory droplets, there are additional risks of airborne spread (less than 5 µm) of nCoV during aerosol generating procedures in ICU and other settings.[6,7] Aerosol-generating procedures in the ICU include: Endotracheal intubation, bronchoscopy, open suctioning, administration of nebulized treatment, bag and mask ventilation, active proning of the patient, disconnecting the patient from the ventilator, non-invasive positive pressure ventilation, tracheostomy, and cardiopulmonary resuscitation. Hence, the patients should ideally be treated in isolation rooms with a functional anteroom for the purpose of donning and doffing of personal protective equipment (PPE). Owing to practical limitations, however, patients may be reasonably isolated in cohorts.

Standard precautions comprise hand hygiene; use of PPE to avoid direct contact with blood, body fluids, secretions (including respiratory secretions) and non-intact skin of the patient; prevention of needle-stick or sharps injury; safe waste management; cleaning and disinfection of equipment and environment. The COVID-19 patients should be exclusively cared by the trained and dedicated healthcare staff who do not have access to other non-COVID-19 patients. The number of people visiting at bedside should be kept to as minimal as needed; the visits by family and relatives should be duly restricted as well. The ICU staff must strictly adhere to the basic infection control measures, viz. hand hygiene, proper use of PPE, disinfection, cleaning and biomedical waste disposal. The healthcare workers should undergo regular structured training regarding the IPC principles. A correct PPE comprises an impervious gown, gloves, tightly fitting mask (FFP2 or FFP3 or respirator in case of strong exposure to aerosols, e.g. endotracheal intubation or bronchoscopy), goggles and a face shield.

INDICATIONS OF ICU ADMISSION

1. **Severe illness**
   - Respiratory rate ≥30 per minute
   - Oxygen saturation at rest ≤93%
   - PaO_2/FiO_2 ≤300 mmHg
2. **Critical/life-threatening illness**
   - Respiratory failure requiring mechanical ventilation
   - Sepsis or septic shock
   - Multiorgan dysfunction syndrome

Requirement of either invasive ventilator support or haemodynamic support with vasoactive agents or both remain the main criteria for ICU admission in a resource-limited setting. Specific triage criteria can be framed for ICU admission based on the framework of institutional protocols.[8] Wherever feasible, the risks, benefits and likelihood of possible outcomes of different treatment options must be discussed with the patients or their care-providers so that they can make informed decisions regarding the institution and continuation of the treatment. In addition to the conventional intensive care wisdom, the treatment should be modified according to the updated scientific guidance from reputed statutory bodies and emerging scientific data on treating COVID-19. The patients in ICU must be assessed regularly (at least every 48 hours) by a multidisciplinary team and the intensive care treatment should be planned and revised accordingly depending on the clinical status of the patient and response to the treatment.

The patient may be discharged from the ICU, if extubated (or spontaneously breathing through tracheostomy) and haemodynamic and oxygenation have stabilized.

The treatment may be stopped compassionately with discussion with the patient, family or the caregivers, if the treatment fails to achieve the overall desired goals and there is little or no likelihood of benefit with continued ICU treatment.

PATHOPHYSIOLOGY OF MULTIORGAN FAILURE (Fig. 9.1)

Upon invasion through the respiratory mucosa, nCoV infects other cells as well and hence results in a systemic cytokine storm. Therefore, a few patients may eventually develop adult respiratory distress syndrome (ARDS), disseminated intravascular coagulation (DIC), septic shock and multiorgan failure.[2] The three core pathologic processes as a result of dysregulated immune system that lead to multiorgan failure and death in COVID-19 are as follows:

1. **Hyperinflammation (cytokine storm):** It is due to aberrant T lymphocyte activation.
2. **Hypercoagulability (increased clotting):** Owing to the endothelial damage and activation of coagulation cascade, it leads to the formation of micro- and macro-blood clots and impaired blood flow.
3. **Severe hypoxaemia (low blood oxygen levels):** The lung inflammation caused by the cytokine storm and microthrombosis in the pulmonary circulation severely impairs oxygen absorption, resulting in oxygenation failure.

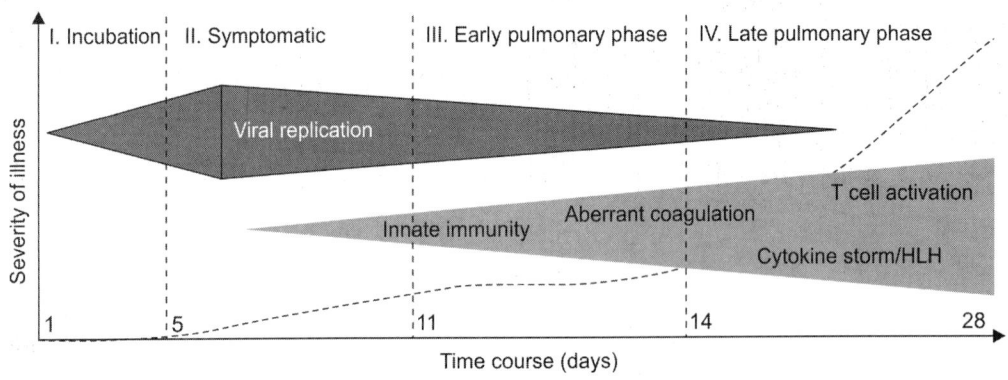

Fig. 9.1: The clinical course of COVID-19 (*Source:* evms.edu/covidcare)

LABORATORY INVESTIGATIONS

1. **Complete blood count:** Lymphopenia, leukopenia (in one-third of patients); thrombocytopenia.
2. **D-dimers:** Elevated.
3. **Procalcitonin (PCT):** Usually normal; may be increased, if associated with a bacterial superinfection.
4. **C-reactive protein (CRP):** Usually elevated; very high values correlate with poor outcomes.
5. **Lactate dehydrogenase (LDH):** Increased in approximately 40% of patients; unspecific LDH $\geq$ 400 IU/ml indicates severe illness.
6. **Troponin:** Increased.

Radiological Imaging

1. **Chest radiograph (CXR):** Shows bilateral infiltrates.
2. **Computed tomography (CT):** Can reveal typical bilateral subpleural ground glass opacities in early stages; should be used when absolutely indicated due to potential risks to healthcare staff and patients.
3. **Ultrasonography:** Should be preferred as a bedside imaging.

TREATMENT

Specific Treatment

With careful risk-benefit evaluation, several drugs with their unique mechanism of actions have been considered as a compassionate use or approved research protocols.

Antiviral Drugs

There is lack of enough data to date to advise a specific antiviral treatment with confirmed efficacy for COVID-19.

a. *Fabiravir and ribavirin:* These are the typical nucleoside analogues that exert a broad-spectrum antiviral effect by lethal mutagenesis, chain termination and inhibition of nucleotide biosynthesis. The combination of fabiravir and oseltamivir has been shown to improve clinical recovery in severe influenza than oseltamivir alone.[9] The combination of ribavirin and interferon-α (IFN-α) has been reported to reduce the 14-day mortality of critically ill MERS and SARS patients.[10] However, their use in the treatment of COVID-19 patients need further evaluation.[11]

b. *Lopinavir/ritonavir:* As a protease inhibitor, the combination is used in the treatment of HIV infection. Lopinavir/ritonavir reveals a promising antiviral activity by inhibiting the replication of coronavirus *in vitro*. Reportedly, the combination of lopinavir/ritonavir and ribavirin could reduce the risk of ARDS compared with ribavirin alone.[12] Owing to serious adverse effects and inconsistent results, further trials are needed.[13]

The combination can be considered in a laboratory-confirmed symptomatic case of COVID-19 at a dose of (400/100 mg) twice daily for 14 days or for 7 days after becoming asymptomatic, provided the following criteria are met:

i. Presence of hypoxaemia or hypotension

ii. High-risk patients (elderly >60 years, diabetes mellitus, chronic pulmonary disease or immunocompromised state)

iii. Presence of ≥1 new onset organ dysfunction

    a. Increase in serum creatinine by 50% from baseline or reduction of glomerular filtration rate (GFR) by ≥25% or urine output <0.5 ml/kg for 6 hours

    b. Decrease of Glasgow Come Scale (GCS) by ≥2

    c. Any other organ dysfunction

c. *Remdesivir (GS-5734):* It is a new potential nucleoside analogue that has antiviral activity against SARS/MERS-CoV and Ebola virus infection.[14] It potentially inhibits the RNA-dependent RNA polymerase, decreases viral replication and improves the recovery of lung parenchyma.[15,16] The combination of remdesivir and IFN-α has been discovered to be better than combination of lopinavir/ritonavir and IFN-α against MERS-CoV.[17] Moreover, the prolonged use of remdesivir in the treatment of Ebola virus infection has been found to be safe.[18]

d. *Umifenovir (arbidol):* It is an indole-derivative small antiviral molecule that has been used for the prophylaxis and treatment of influenza and other respiratory viral infections.[19] It may inhibit viral entry into the cells and stimulate immune response.[20] The efficacy of its derivative—arbidol mesylate was approximately five times higher than the parent compound in reducing the reproduction of SARS in cells *in vitro*.[21] Clinical trials have shown promising results in patients with nCoV.[22,23]

Antimalarial Drugs

By binding to the spike (S) protein of the virus, the angiotensin-converting enzyme 2 (ACE2), a membrane protein that acts as a functional receptor of SARS-CoV, can facilitate the entry of virus into the cells through the fusion of viral and host cell membranes.[24-26] It appears, therefore, logically appealing to block the binding of S protein to attenuate viral infection.[27]

a. *Chloroquine:* Chloroquine, as sulphate and phosphate salts, is a 9-aminoquinoline has been clinically used for the treatment of malaria and various autoimmune diseases. Due to its inhibitory effect on ACE2, it exerts broad-spectrum antiviral properties and may potentially inhibit SARS-CoV infection.[28,29] As the nCoV enters the epithelial cells of oral mucosa essentially via the ACE2 receptor, chloroquine can exert its effects at entry as well as post-entry stages of infection.[30] Wang et al have demonstrated the efficacy of chloroquine in nCoV infection *in vitro*.[31] In another study involving more than 100 COVID-19 patients, chloroquine has been superior to the control treatment in clinical and radiological improvement of pneumonia, shortening the course of the disease and improving virus negative conversion.[32]

b. *Hydroxychloroquine:* It is a 4-aminoquinoline derivative antimalarial drug. Due to its immunosuppressive properties, it has been used in diseases such as rheumatoid arthritis (RA) and systemic lupus erythematosus (SLE).[33,34] Being more potent than chloroquine in producing *in vitro* inhibition of nCoV, hydroxychloroquine has been administered for the treatment of COVID-19 as 400 mg twice daily for day 1, followed by 200 mg twice daily for next 4 days.[35]

Adjunctive Treatment

The effect of nCov on the human immune system depends on several factors. In patients with normal immune system, the viral infection may activate the immune cells and create a state of cytokine storm which manifests as disease severity.[36] On the contrary, the elderly and patients with chronic diseases have low lymphocytic counts, particularly CD4+ cells, and consequently a deficient immune system. Therefore, a wide variety of pharmacological agents have been attempted to optimally modulate the immune responses.[37,38]

1. *Corticosteroids:* The use to systemic corticosteroids for the treatment of viral pneumonia or ARDS remains controversial. While immunomodulation with high-dose methylprednisolone regimen may attenuate inflammatory response and parenchymal damage,[39,40] use of steroids promotes opportunistic bacterial and

fungal infections, causes avascular necrosis, increases blood sugar levels, produces psychosis, increases mortality, decreases viral clearance and even tends to promote antiviral resistance.[41–44] Similarly, corticosteroid treatment in patients with MERS did not reveal any difference in mortality, but was associated with delayed MERS coronavirus RNA clearance.[45] The early administration of parenteral steroids for the reduction in fever and prevention of pneumonia has been found to increase mortality from H1N1 infection.[46] Hence, steroids cannot be routinely advised in patients with ARDS.[47] Research in SARS and influenza has failed to reveal any benefit for patients treated with steroids. However, low-dose hydrocortisone may be indicated in septic shock refractory to fluids and vasopressors.[48]

2. *Tocilizumab:* The cytokine storm in COVID-19 is marked by elevated levels of interleukin-6 (IL-6), IFN-α and other cytokines that lead to ARDS and multiple organ failure.[49] Tocilizumab is a recombinant monoclonal antibody that binds to IL-6 and inhibits its signal transduction. It has been used in treatment of rheumatoid arthritis (RA) and in the management of cytokine release syndrome induced by chimeric antigen receptor T cell (CAR-T) infusion against B cell acute lymphoblastic leukaemia.[50,51] Tocilizumab has been recommended for the immunotherapy of patients with extensive lung parenchymal lesions, but its role in nCoV infection needs further evaluation.[52]

3. *Cyclosporin A:* Cyclophilin A, an immunophilin, is the cellular receptor for cyclosporin A. Cyclosporin A, a popular immunosuppressant that is used in transplantation and autoimmune disorders, inhibits cyclophilins and blocks the replication of coronavirus, including nCoV.[53] Its role as a CoV-inhibitor needs further validation.

4. *Thymosin alpha-1:* It is a thymic peptide hormone that significantly restores homeostasis of the host immune system.[54,55] It improves the lymphopenia associated with severe sepsis, decreases mortality and improves clinical outcome.[56] It has also been demonstrated to facilitate enhanced immune response in SARS patients and used to enhance cellular immunity against viral infection.[57]

5. *Interferons:* Out of the two types of interferons (IFNs), type I IFNs have been described to inhibit replication of SARS and MERS CoV.[58,59] Priming with small amounts of IFNs partially restores innate host immunity to SARS-CoV.[60] Combination therapy of IFN-α-2a with ribavirin has been found to improve patient survival in MERS-Cov infection.[59]

6. *Gamma globulin:* Intravenous gamma globulin contains high titres of neutralizing antibodies against multiple pathogens, including viruses and bacteria and has been used in the treatment of severe infection and sepsis; however, the mortality benefit has not been established.[61,62]

7. *Convalescent plasma:* The convalescent plasma derived from the patients with antibodies against nCov can reduce the mortality rate of critically ill COVID-19 patients.[63] It has been demonstrated to be effective in the past for the treatment of SARS, MES and Ebola virus disease.[64–66] It is presumed that the antibodies from convalescent plasma might decrease viraemia and improve the lung parenchymal damage.[67,68]

Antibacterial Treatment

Although a prophylactic antibiotic is not indicated, an empiric broad-spectrum antibiotic therapy should be initiated as early as possible (preferably within 1 hour) in a patient suspected to have a bacterial infection as there is a high incidence of bacterial coinfection or cross-infection for critically ill COVID-19 patients. It is recommended to obtain blood (and other suitable) cultures prior to the initiation of empiric antimicrobial therapy; however, antimicrobial therapy should not be unduly delayed to collect blood cultures. Empirical therapy with antimicrobials should be administered, in addition to antiviral therapy, in COVID-19 patients: (i) who have initial severe manifestations (e.g. extensive pneumonia, respiratory failure, hypotension and febrile illness), or (ii) who deteriorate after initial improvement, or (iii) who do not show any sign of improvement on after 3 to 5 days of antiviral therapy.[69] The choice of empiric antibiotic should be based on the clinical diagnosis and local antibiogram. It should be regularly evaluated and de-escalated depending on the culture and sensitivity results or clinical decision. Evaluation of serum PCT and CRP may aid timely diagnosis and treatment of bacterial infection.

MANAGEMENT OF HYPOXAEMIC RESPIRATORY FAILURE AND ADULT RESPIRATORY DISTRESS SYNDROME (ARDS)

Although the exact incidence of hypoxic respiratory failure in patients with COVID-19 needs to be determined, it seems that around 14% will develop severe disease requiring oxygen therapy, and 5% will require ICU admission and mechanical ventilation.[1] Severe hypoxaemic respiratory failure is suspected when a patient with respiratory distress is failing standard oxygen therapy, i.e. when oxygen is delivered via a face mask with reservoir bag (flow rates of 10–15 l/min; FiO_2 0.60–0.95). Hypoxaemic respiratory failure in ARDS commonly results from intrapulmonary ventilation/perfusion (V/Q) mismatch or shunt. Risk factors associated with respiratory failure requiring mechanical ventilation include older age (>60 years), male gender, and the presence of underlying comorbidities such as diabetes mellitus, malignancy, and immunocompromised state.[70]

The onset of ARDS is characterized by new or worsening respiratory symptoms within a week of known clinical insult. ARDS is defined as acute breathlessness (>7 to 10 days) with the following characteristics:

1. $PaO_2/FiO_2 \leq 300$ mmHg (or $SpO_2/FiO_2 \leq 315$, when PaO_2 is not available)
2. Bilateral (patchy, diffuse, or homogeneous) infiltrates consistent with pulmonary oedema
3. No clinical evidence of left atrial hypertension

In a non-ventilated patient or patient on mechanical ventilation with PEEP or CPAP ≥ 5 cm H_2O, ARDS is classified based on PaO_2/FiO_2 ratio.

Type	PaO_2/FiO_2(mmHg)
1. Mild	200–300
2. Moderate	100–200
3. Severe	<100

Respiratory Supportive Strategies

Owing to high incidence of hypoxaemia, ARDS and respiratory failure in critically ill COVID-19 patients, institution of timely and effective respiratory support can reduce complications and improve their survival to an extent.[71]

Oxygen Therapy, High-Flow Nasal Cannula and Non-Invasive Ventilation

The adequacy of oxygenation should be ascertained, and supplemental oxygen should be administered immediately at a rate of 5 l/min in patients with hypoxaemia, respiratory distress and shock. Oxygen therapy, high-flow nasal cannula (HFNC), and non-invasive ventilation (NIV) may lessen the need of endotracheal intubation and mechanical ventilation and thus minimize the associated complications and mortality. In adults with COVID-19 and acute hypoxaemic respiratory failure on supplemental oxygen, the target SpO_2 should be ≥90% in non-pregnant individuals and ≥92–95% in pregnant adults. Single-use, disposable oxygen-delivery interfaces, such as nasal cannula, simple face mask or mask with reservoir bag, should be used.

If the conventional oxygen therapy fails to improve the acute hypoxaemic respiratory failure, use of HFNC (with the patient's face covered with a surgical mask) as an alternative to NIV may be considered. HFNC can deliver 60 l/min of gas flow (around 15 l/min for paediatric circuits) and an FiO_2 up to 1.0 in adults. Although it may decrease the need for endotracheal intubation, it should be avoided in hypercapnic states (e.g. exacerbation of chronic obstructive pulmonary disease, pulmonary oedema), haemodynamic instability, multiple organ failure or altered mental status. HFNC has been demonstrated to significantly decrease 90-day mortality of community-acquired pneumonia compared with standard oxygen or NIV.[72] It has been demonstrated by Hui et al that the breath dispersion distance is limited, thereby reducing the risk of airborne transmission.[73] However, oxygen supplementation through HFNC and NIV may generate aerosol and increase the risk of virus transmission to the healthcare staff. Hence, it must be ensured that HFNC and NIV systems have good interface fitting, as any loose connection of the cannula with nasal obstruction can significantly increase the dispersion distance. It is also imperative, therefore, on the part of the medical personnel at bedside to wear appropriate N95 masks and stringently adhere PPE guidelines to contain nosocomial transmission.[74,75] Although various studies have quoted the failure rate of NIV to be as high as 85% in the treatment of severe influenzas A (H1N1),[76] it may be effective in selected patients with early and mild acute hypoxaemic respiratory failure.[77] NIV risks delayed/emergent intubation, large tidal volumes and high transpulmonary pressures. NIV with a helmet should be preferred, if available.

It is rather prudent to be restrictive with HFNC and NIV in the setting of COVID-19. There should be constant monitoring for any worsening respiratory status and oxygen index (PaO_2/FiO_2 ratio) of the patient, and mechanical ventilation should never be unduly delayed. In patients with severe hypoxaemia (PaO_2/FiO_2 ≤200/mmHg), early intubation and invasive mechanical ventilation should be considered. Any kind of deliberate or otherwise postponement of intubation in patients failing NIV worsens outcome; likewise, any emergency intubation in COVID-19 patients puts healthcare staff at risk and should be best avoided.

Intubation, Mechanical Ventilation and other Procedures

Owing to the risk of aerosol formation, various airway procedures (e.g. endotracheal intubation, bronchoscopy, open suction, bag ventilation and tracheostomy) should only be performed, if absolutely necessary and appropriate airborne precautions must be observed (use of PPE including FFP2/FFP3 masks, goggles and face shields). The airway intervention procedures should preferably be performed by the most experienced personnel with a wide expertise and skills in airway management in order to minimize the number of attempts and risk of transmission. Patients with ARDS, particularly children, obese and pregnant, may desaturate rapidly during intubation. Preoxygenation with 100% FiO_2 for 5 minutes should be performed via a face mask with reservoir bag, bag-valve mask, HFNC or NIV can be performed. A rapid sequence induction without intermittent bag mask ventilation should be preferred, if possible, so as to reduce aerosol formation.[78] Use of a videolaryngoscope for intubation may help to safely increase the distance between the anaesthesiologist and the patient, and, if available, should be preferred over direct laryngoscopy.[79] Confirmation of correct placement of endotracheal tube can be done bydirect visualization or capnography; use of the stethoscope for auscultation of breath sounds should be avoided.

Regarding aerosol-generating procedures, viz. tracheal intubation, bronchoscopies, or non-invasive positive pressure ventilation, the WHO guidance on COVID-19 recommends the use of negative pressure rooms with a minimum of 12 air changes per hour or at least 160 l/second/patient in facilities with natural ventilation.[80] Bronchoscopic procedures tend to produce the maximal risk of aerosolization, and hence should only be used cautiously when indicated. For invasive ventilation, use of closed inline suction catheters are advisable. Any disconnection of the patient from the ventilatory circuit should be avoided as far as practical to avoid decruitment of the lungs and aerosolization; for any intended circuit disconnection, the endotracheal tube should be clamped and the ventilator disabled to prevent aerosolization. Use of nebulizers is not recommended and metered dose inhalers (MDI) should be preferred where possible.

While non-invasive ventilation in select patients with mild ARDS may be attempted, but one should have a low threshold for early intubation, preferably with an endotracheal (ET) tube with subglottic suction. Patients with ARDS should be ventilated with ARDS net protocol. Mechanical ventilation is a potentially life-saving intervention, but it can promote lung injury and contribute to multiorgan failure.[81]

Mechanical ventilation for patients with severe ARDS should be managed with lung-protective strategies to minimize ventilator-associated lung injury and to improve survival, viz. ventilation with low tidal volumes (4 to 8 ml/kg of predicted body weight), targeting plateau pressure (<30 cm H_2O) and minimizing the inspired oxygen concentration to decrease oxygen toxicity.[82] Tidal volume up to 8 ml/kg PBW may be allowed, if undesirable adverse effects, such as ventilator dyssynchrony or pH 7.15 occur. Hypercapnia is permissible as long as the target pH is within the range of 7.30 to 7.45. Deep sedation may be needed to control the respiratory drive and achieve the targeted tidal volume. High driving pressures (i.e. the difference between plateau pressure and PEEP) may be more reliable predictor of increased mortality in ARDS than high tidal volume or plateau pressure.

i. *Steps in ventilator set-up and adjustment*
   1. Calculate predicted body weight (PBW).
      - Males = 50 + 2.3 [height (inches)—60].
      - Females = 45.5 + 2.3 [height (inches)—60].
   2. Select volume A/C mode on the ventilator.
   3. Set ventilator settings to achieve initial tidal volume (VT)= 6 ml/kg PBW.
   4. Set initial respiratory rate (RR) to approximate baseline minute ventilation (not >35 bpm).
   5. Aim for a pH over 7.2, no need to fear about the $PaCO_2$ (permissive hypercapnia).
   6. If the $PaCO_2$ level rises too much in spite of a respiratory rate (RR) of 35, try to reduce the dead space in the circuit.
   7. If the pH drops below 7.2, consider adding sodium bicarbonate infusion.
   8. Adjust VT and RR to achieve pH and plateau pressure goals as mentioned below.
ii. *Oxygenation goal:* PaO_2 55–80 mmHg or oxygen saturation (SpO_2) 88–95%
   1. Use a minimum positive end expiratory pressure (PEEP) of 5 cm H_2O. Consider the use of incremental FiO_2/PEEP combinations as shown below to achieve the goal.
   2. Plateau pressure goal: ≤30 cm H_2O
   3. Check Pplat (0.5 second inspiratory pause) at least every 4 hours and after each change in PEEP or VT.
   4. If the Pplat remains above 30 cm H_2O, decrease VT by 1 ml/kg steps (minimum = 4 ml/kg).
iii. *Fluid management:* Use a conservative fluid management strategy for ARDS patients without tissue hypoperfusion.[83]

High positive end-expiratory pressure (PEEP) decreases the need for high FiO_2 by improving gas exchange and lung compliance, whereas too high PEEP may lead to lung overdistension and haemodynamic instability. Optimal PEEP can be titrated by pressure–volume curve, oxygenation, stress index, electrical impedance tomography (EIT), ultrasound, and some other clinical parameters. In patients with moderate or severe ARDS, higher PEEP strategy is preferred instead of lower PEEP. PEEP titration requires a considerable balance between the potential merits (reduced atelectrauma and improved alveolar recruitment) and the demerits (end-inspiratory overdistension leading to lung injury and higher pulmonary vascular resistance). Lung recruitment needs to be evaluated for mechanically ventilated patients when uncorrectable hypoxaemia occurs, and lung recruitment should be executed for patients whose lungs can restore aeration. CT, EIT, ultrasound, and other bedside techniques should be used to evaluate lung recruitability before lung recruitment. For mechanically ventilated adults with moderate to severe ARDS, intermittent boluses of neuromuscular blocking agents (NMBA) may be administered to control the spontaneous breathing and facilitate protective lung ventilation. In certain situations, viz. persistent ventilator dyssynchrony, need for ongoing deep sedation, prone ventilation, or persistently high plateau pressures, a continuous NMBA infusion for up to 48 hours may be considered. The routine use of inhaled nitric oxide is not recommended.

Prone Positioning

COVID-19 may lead to acute respiratory distress syndrome (ARDS), necessitating invasive mechanical ventilation with lung protective lung ventilation. Despite these measures, some ARDS patients develop refractory hypoxaemia.[84] Therefore, in patients with moderate to severe ARDS failing conventional supine mechanical ventilation, prone positioning for 12 to 16 hours may be considered. Prone positioning, as a simple intervention, improves oxygenation and increases bronchial secretion clearance. It neither requires any specialised equipment nor entails any additional cost (except trained human resources); hence it can be implemented in low- and middle-income settings. Prone positioning, passive (conscious) or active, can be applied to all critically ill patients. This strategy has been associated with decreased ventilator-induced lung injury and increased survival in patients with severe acute respiratory distress syndrome (ARDS) with refractory hypoxaemia.[85,86]

Prone positioning ventilation often improves oxygenation in ARDS through improvements in ventilation/perfusion matching, the uniformity of ventilation, and gravity-related atelectasis. Although prone ventilation has been used in mechanically ventilated SARS patients, but the results were inconclusive.[71] However, several other studies demonstrated improved oxygenation, decreased carbon dioxide retention and decreased mortality with early application of prone positioning in patients with severe ARDS.[84,87] Prone positioning has multiple physiological benefits:[88,89]

1. **Improved VQ mismatch** (increased PaO_2 secondary to better homogeneous aeration of lungs and enhancing the ventral-dorsal transpulmonary pressure gradient.)

2. **Reduced shunt** (while the perfusion pattern remains relatively unchanged, the lung aeration becomes more homogenous.)

3. **Recruitment of the posterior lung segments** (as the result of reversal of atelectasis)

4. **Increased clearance of respiratory secretions**

However, prone positioning may lead to displacement of vascular lines and endotracheal tube, increases the risk of pressure sores, facial oedema, corneal abrasions and brachial plexus injury and cause transient haemodynamic instability. Healthcare workers involved in proning COVID-19 patients should be well-trained in the appropriate proning technique and infection control precautions. It should be avoided in patients with unstable spine or open abdominal or thoracic trauma. Therefore, prone ventilation is a relatively safe procedure that can be recommended for the treatment of 2019-nCoV-induced severe ARDS.

Extracorporeal Life Support (ECLS)

Extracorporeal life support (or extracorporeal memberane oxygenation, ECMO) is a supportive care strategy to optimize oxygenation and ventilation in patients with potentially reversible severe ARDS with hypoxaemia and/or hypercapnia that is refractory to conventional treatment.[90] Observational studies have shown that use of ECMO lowers hospital mortality in patients with ARDS induced by H1N1 infuenza and MERS.[91,92]

Where available, the decision to institute venovenous ECMO should not be delayed in severe ARDS and refractory hypoxaemia (PaO_2/FiO_2 <80 mmHg) patients with failed lung recruitment and prone positioning. Moreover, COVID-19 patients may need ECMO support for cardiac arrhythmias or shock. However, ECMO may not be very useful in patients with septic shock and multiple organ failure.[93] As ECMO is a resource-intensive, highly specialized and expensive technique with potential for major complications, viz. haemorrhage and nosocomial infection, hence it should be used judiciously in the treatment of COVID-19.[94]

HAEMODYNAMIC SUPPORT AND MANAGEMENT OF SEPTIC SHOCK

Estimated incidence of shock in COVID-19 patients admitted in ICU may up to reach 20–35%. Myocardial injury, i.e. elevation of cardiac biomarkers, has also been reported in COVID-19 patients.[5,36,93] The risk factors for haemodynamic instability in COVID-19 patients are old age, comorbidities (especially diabetes and cardiovascular disease including hypertension), lower lymphocyte count, higher D-dimer level, and possible myocardial injury. Septic shock is a possibility, if an infection is suspected or confirmed, vasopressors are needed to maintain mean arterial pressure (MAP) ≥65 mmHg and serum lactate is ≥2 mmol/l, provided hypovolaemia is ruled out. Standard care includes early administration of empiric antimicrobial therapy, fluid loading and start of vasopressors. In adults, administration of at least 30 ml/kg of isotonic crystalloid should be done. Hypotonic crystalloids, starches, or gelatines should be avoided. If there is no response to fluid loading and signs of volume overload begin to appear (e.g. jugular venous distension or presence of crepts on lung auscultation), fluid administration should be discontinued. Additional fluid boluses (250–1000 ml in adults) may be needed based on clinical response and improvement of perfusion targets. Perfusion targets include MAP >65 mmHg, urine output (>0.5 ml/kg/h in adults) and improvement of skin mottling, level of consciousness and serum lactate, and increased capillary refill. The dynamic indices of volume responsiveness include passive leg raises, serial stroke volume measurements, or variations in systolic pressure, pulse pressure, inferior vena cava size, or stroke volume in response to changes in intrathoracic pressure during mechanical ventilation. Hypotonic solutions are less effective at increasing intravascular volume. Vasopressors need to be administered when shock persists during or after fluid resuscitation. The initial blood pressure target is MAP ≥65 mmHg in adults. If central venous access is not available, vasopressors can be given through a peripheral vein provided a large vein is used and there are no signs of extravasation and local tissue necrosis. Vasopressors can also be administered through intraosseous needles.

The use of dynamic assessment to guide fluid therapy was found to reduce mortality.[95] Compared with central venous oxygen saturation (ScvO$_2$) guided therapy, early lactate clearance-directed therapy was associated with a reduction in mortality and shorter duration of mechanical ventilation.[96] Besides hypovolaemia, an increased serum lactate level may indicate mitochondrial dysfunction, liver failure, mesenteric ischaemia, or epinephrine infusion. In the ANDROMEDA-SHOCK trial, capillary refill testing (CRT) every 30 min was associated with a non-significant reduction in mortality compared with serum lactate measurement every 2 hours.[97] For the acute resuscitation of adults with COVID-19 and shock, an initial conservative approach to fluid resuscitation, preferably with buffered/balanced crystalloids is advisable. With limited availability of buffered solutions, however, 0.9% saline remains a reasonable alternative. The routine use of albumin for initial resuscitation is not recommended. Aggressive fluid resuscitation may negatively impact oxygenation.

Vasoactive Agents

Norepinephrine as the first-line vasoactive agent is preferred. If norepinephrine is not available, either vasopressin or epinephrine may be used. While digital ischaemia may occur with the use of vasopressin, epinephrine may cause tachycardia and excess lactate production. Dopamine should be avoided due to the inherent risk of arrhythmias. Adding vasopressin as a second-line agent may be an option, if target MAP cannot be achieved by norepinephrine alone. A target MAP of 60–65 mmHg should be considered. For adults with COVID-19 with evidence of myocardial dysfunction and persistent hypoperfusion despite fluid resuscitation and norepinephrine administration, addition of dobutamine may be a prudent option rather than increasing norepinephrine dose. For adults' refractory shock, low-dose corticosteroid therapy may be considered (shock-reversal).

RENAL REPLACEMENT THERAPY

For a COVID-19 patient, the renal support can be provided by use of 7–14 hours of prolonged intermittent renal replacement therapy (PIRRT) via continuous venovenous haemodiafiltration (CVVDHF) so as to limit staff interactions. Systemic anticoagulation can be initiated by administration of unfractionated heparin as 80 units/kg IV bolus, followed by a 1000 units/h IV infusion, the target aPTT is 60–80, and should be checked after 6 hours of initiating the treatment and titrated accordingly.

NUTRITION THERAPY

The nutritional management of the COVID-19 patient is principally similar to any other ICU patient admitted with pulmonary compromise regarding timing, route, and monitoring of nutritional therapy.

Nutrition Assessment

Majority of the critically ill COVID-19 patients have negative nitrogen balance and malnutrition that acts as a contributing risk factor to the emergence of viral infectious diseases.[2,36]

Timing of Nutrition Delivery

Early enteral nutrition (EN) should be started within 24–36 hours of admission to the ICU or within 12 hours of intubation and initiation of mechanical ventilation as it improves mortality and reduces the likelihood of infections in ICU.[98–100]

Route, Tube Placement and Method of Nutrition Delivery

EN is preferred to parenteral nutrition (PN) and the majority of patients with sepsis or septic shock tolerate early EN at a trophic rate.[101] A large bore nasogastric (NGT) or orogastric (OGT) tube may be placed at time of intubation and its confirmation via abdominal X-rays should be clustered with chest X-ray timing so as to optimise resource utilization. Placement of an enteral access device is an aerosol-generating procedure. If gastric feeding is not tolerated, a prokinetic agent may be added or a bedside placement of post-pyloric EN delivery is advised. Post-pyloric feeding tubes tend to be smaller in caliber and may often become clogged. As time taken for the placement of post-pyloric feeding tubes may be longer than that for the gastric tubes, possibility of an increased exposure time of the healthcare staff should be considered. Continuous rather than bolus EN is advisable.

Early PN should be started in the high-risk patients (e.g. need of escalating or multiple vasopressors, high ventilatory support or rising serum lactate levels) for whom early gastric EN is not feasible. EN may be restarted after achieving adequate resuscitation and a sustained mean arterial pressure of >65 mmHg on a stable vasopressor dose.[102] Although the incidence of bowel ischaemia in shock is around 0.3%, it may be a concern for COVID-19 patients where prolonged ICU stay is expected. Early PN helps reduce the occurrence of bowel ischaemia, and in addition, also minimises the droplet or aerosol transmission to healthcare staff by evading the necessity of placement of an enteral access device. In COVID-19 patients with gastrointestinal (GI) involvement, such as diarrhoea, nausea, vomiting, abdominal discomfort and GI bleeding, early use of PN should be considered; EN feed may be started once the GI symptoms subside.[103–105] PN should also be considered in patients with increasing nasogastric outputs in previous 6 to 12 hours with start of trophic feeds or prior to initiation of EN.[106] Critically ill patients with COVID-19 disease are often at-risk of refeeding syndrome. Therefore, feed should be initiated at approximately 25% of caloric goal in such patients; frequent monitoring of serum phosphate, magnesium and potassium levels should be done as calories are gradually increased.

Nutrition Dose

Feeding should be initiated with low dose EN, defined as hypocaloric or trophic, advancing to full dose EN slowly over the first week of the critical illness to meet an energy goal of 15–20 kcal/kg/day (approximately 70–80% of total caloric requirements) and protein goal of 1.2–2.0 g/kg/day. Likewise, if PN is considered necessary, conservative dextrose content and volume should be used in the early phase of critical illness, slowly advancing to meet the same energy goals as outlined above. Nutrition requirements should take into consideration the use of propofol in terms of lipid calories and total calories needed.

Formula Selection

A standard high protein (>20% protein) polymeric isosmotic enteral formula should be used in the early acute phase of critical illness. Addition of fibre should be considered as the vasopressor requirements decline. In case of a significant GI dysfunction, a fibre-free formula may be better tolerated. COVID-19 patients develop a cytokine storm which resembles secondary haemophagocytic lymphohistiocytosis (HLH), and presence of hypertriglyceridaemia and increasing ferritin, CRP and transaminases may help in the identification of secondary HLH. Treatment of secondary HLH includes high dose methyl prednisolone (120 mg, 8 hourly) for 3 days, followed by weaning as per clinical and laboratory improvement.[107]

Monitoring Nutrition Tolerance

Patients should be monitored by daily physical examination and confirmation of passage of faeces and flatus. Enteral feeding intolerance (EFI) is frequently observed during the early and late acute phases of critical illness in COVID-19 patients. Gastric residual volume monitoring is not reliable for detection of delayed gastric emptying and bears an inherent risk of aspiration and virus transmission to the staff.[108]

Nutrition for the Patient Undergoing Prone Positioning

EN during prone positioning is not associated with increased risk of gastrointestinal or pulmonary complications.[109-111] While most patients tolerate gastric feeds in the prone position, post-pyloric placement of the feeding tube may be indicated occasionally. When EN is administered during prone positioning, the head of the bed should be elevated (reverse Trendelenburg) to at least 10 to 25° to decrease the risk of aspiration of gastric contents, facial oedema and intra-abdominal hypertension.[112]

Nutrition Therapy during ECMO

There is lack of data regarding nutritional support during ECMO in COVID-19 disease. It is often considered that patients put on ECMO are at-risk of delayed gastric emptying and bowel ischaemia.[113] Other observational data shows safety and tolerability of gastric EN delivery during ECMO.[114] Therefore, starting early low dose (trophic) EN with slow advancement to goal over the first week of critical illness in patients on ECMO may be considered with vigilant monitoring for EFI.[115] With PN, the early ECMO filters allowed lipid infiltration into the oxygenator; but the newer ECMO circuits do not pose any such issue.

LABORATORY DIAGNOSIS AND SPECIMENS

Real-time polymerase chain reaction (RT-PCR) is the gold standard for similar viral infections, including nCoV.[116] Notably, COVID-19 poses several diagnostic challenges due to an extended incubation period of almost two weeks that includes a prolonged interval (approximately 5 days) of viral shedding prior to the onset of symptoms. Moreover, the duration of asymptomatic shedding is not only variable, but may also change based on the anatomic level (upper versus lower) of the infection in the respiratory system.[117]

It is recommended to collect specimens from both the upper respiratory tract (URT; nasopharynx and oropharynx) and lower respiratory tract (LRT; expectorated sputum, endotracheal aspirate, or bronchoalveolar lavage) for nCoV testing by RT-PCR. Sputum induction should be avoided due to the risk of aerosol transmission. In mechanically ventilated patients, only LRT samples may be collected, if readily obtainable. Sample should not be obtained from the nostrils or tonsils. Appropriate PPE for specimen collection should be used (droplet and contact precautions for URT specimens and additional airborne precautions for LRT specimens). When collecting URT samples, viral swabs (sterile Dacron or rayon, not cotton) and viral transport media (VTM) should be used.

For intubated and mechanically ventilated adults, lower respiratory tract specimens are considered to give a higher diagnostic yield than upper respiratory (nasopharyngeal or oropharyngeal) specimens in patients with pneumonia, consistent with what was observed for SARS, and should, therefore, be obtained whenever possible.[118]

Moreover, obtaining endotracheal aspirate should be preferred to bronchoalveolar lavage samples. Bronchoalveolar lavage should be limited and performed, only if indicated and with adequate precautions, due to the risk of aerosolization and consequent exposure of healthcare professionals. Similarly, sputum induction should be avoided due to increased risk of aerosolization. Endotracheal aspirate specimens appear to carry a lower risk of aerosolization, and can sometimes be obtained without disconnecting the patient from the ventilator. A single negative swab from the upper airway does not rule out nCoV infection; the swab might turn out to be negative in a later stage, despite the presence of infectious viral shedding in the lower airways. Hence, repeated sampling from multiple sites, including the lower respiratory tract, will increase diagnostic yield.[119]

Owing to high specificity of RT-PCR, a single positive swab confirms the diagnosis of COVID-19 and should be adequate to trigger infection control precautions and appropriate treatment of the patient. In hospitalized patients with confirmed nCoV infection, repeat URT and LRT samples should be collected to establish viral clearance. The frequency of specimen collection will depend on local circumstances, but should be at least every 48 to 96 hours until there are two consecutive negative results (both URT and LRT samples, if both are collected) in a clinically recovered patient at least 24 hours apart.

Given that coinfection with other viral pathogens has been observed, a positive test for another respiratory virus does not rule out COVID-19, and should not delay testing, if there is a high suspicion of COVID-19. Dual infections with other respiratory viral infections have been found in SARS and MERS cases. Both URT and LRT specimens can be tested for other respiratory viruses, such as influenza A and B (including zoonotic influenza A), respiratory syncytial virus, parainfluenza viruses, rhinoviruses, adenoviruses, enteroviruses (e.g. EVD68), human metapneumovirus, and endemic human coronaviruses (i.e. HKU1, OC43, NL63, and 229E). LRT specimens can also be tested for bacterial pathogens, including *Legionella pneumophila*.

PREVENTION OF COMPLICATIONS

1. **Lessen the days of invasive mechanical ventilation**
   i. Use weaning protocols, daily assess the patient for readiness to breathe spontaneously.
   ii. Reduce continuous or intermittent sedation by targeting specific titration endpoints (light sedation, unless contraindicated) or with daily interruption of continuous sedative infusions.
2. **Decrease incidence of ventilator-associated pneumonia**
   i. Prefer oral intubation to nasal intubation in adults.
   ii. Keep patient in semirecumbent position (head of bed elevation 30–45°).
   iii. Use a closed suctioning system; periodically drain and discard condensate in tubing.
   iv. Use a new ventilator circuit for each patient; do not routinely change circuit (change it, only if it is soiled or damaged).
   v. Change heat moisture exchanger (HME) when it malfunctions, when soiled, or every 5–7 days.

3. **Reduce incidence of venous thromboembolism:** Use pharmacological prophylaxis {low molecular-weight heparin (LMWH, preferred) or heparin 5000 units subcutaneously twice daily} in adults without contraindications. For those with contraindications, use mechanical prophylaxis such as intermittent pneumatic compression devices.

4. **Reduce incidence of catheter-related bloodstream infection** (CRBSI): Use a checklist for sterile insertion and as a daily reminder to remove catheter, if no longer needed.

5. **Reduce incidence of pressure ulcers:** Frequent turning the position of the patient (e.g. every 2 hours).

6. **Reduce incidence of stress ulcers and gastrointestinal bleeding**
   i. Start early enteral nutrition (within 24–48 hours of admission).
   ii. Administer histamine-2 receptor blockers or proton-pump inhibitors in patients with risk factors for GI bleeding (e.g. mechanical ventilation for $\geq$48 hours, coagulopathy, renal replacement therapy, liver disease, multiple comorbidities, and higher organ failure score).

7. **Reduce incidence of ICU-related weakness**
   i. Avoid neuromuscular blocking agents as far as possible.
   ii. Attempt active early mobilization of the patient, if safe.

SUMMARY

As there is lack of specific antiviral therapy or vaccines for COVID-19 at present, it is essential to augment the host immune response against the infection. Most of the treatment strategies are based on our understanding gained during treating the recent infections of SARS, MERS, Ebola or some other previous influenza viruses. There is no current scientific evidence from randomized control trials (RCTs) to recommend any specific line of treatment against nCoV. Hence, the efficacy of existing pharmacological agents and other adjunctive interventions need further clinical validation. Till then, the practice of vigilant intensive care monitoring, appropriate application of respiratory supportive strategies, pharmacological and non-pharmacological support of multiple organ function, modulating the immune status and inflammatory responses, prevention of complications and reducing secondary infection are crucial for the smooth and successful recovery of critically ill COVID-19 patients. We need to contemplate, find the problems, address the critical issues to be improved, establish a database, promote research and constantly endeavour for the advancement of the critical care discipline.

REFERENCES

1. Wu Z, McGoogan JM. Characteristics of important lessons from the coronavirus disease 2019 (COVID-19) outbreak in China: Summary of a report of 72/314 cases from the Chinese Center for Disease Control and Prevention. JAMA 2020;323(13):1239–42.

2. Sun P, MD Qie S, Liu Z, Ren J, Li K, Xi J. Clinical characteristics of 50466 patients with 2019-nCoV infection. J Med Virol 2020. doi: 2020. https://doi.org/10.1002/jmv.25735

3. Arabi YM, Fowler R, Hayden FG. Critical care management of adults with community-acquired severe respiratory viral infection. Intensive Care Med 2020;46(2):315–28. doi: 10.1007/s00134-020-05943-5

4. Wang Z, Chen, X, Lu Y, Chen F, Zhang W. Clinical characteristics and therapeutic procedure for four cases with 2019 novel coronavirus pneumonia receiving combined Chinese and Western medicine treatment. Biosci Trends 2020;14(1):64–68.

5. Yang X, Yu Y, Xu J, et al. Clinical course and outcomes of critically ill patients with SARS-CoV-2 pneumonia in Wuhan, China: a single-centered, retrospective, observational study. Lancet Respir Med 2020; S2213-2600(20)30079-5. doi:10.1016/S2213-2600(20)30079–5

6. Yu YX, Sun L, Yao K, Lou XT, Liang X, Zhao BW, Mu QX, Du H, Zhao Y, Zhang H. Consideration and prevention for the aerosol transmission of 2019 novel coronavirus. Zhonghua Yan Ke Za Zhi 2020;56(0):E008. doi: 10.3760/cma.j.cn112142-20200313-00181

7. van Doremalen N, Bushmaker T, Morris DH, Holbrook MG, Gamble A, Williamson BN, Tamin A, Harcourt JL, Thornburg NJ, Gerber SI, Lloyd-Smith JO, de Wit E, Munster VJ. N Engl J Med 2020; 382:1564-1567. doi: 10.1056/NEJMc2004973.

8. Swiss Med Wkly. 2020;150:w20229

9. Wang Y, Fan G, Salam A, et al. Comparative effectiveness of combined favipiravir and oseltamivir therapy versus oseltamivir monotherapy in critically ill patients with infuenza virus infection. J Infect Dis 2019. https://doi.org/10.1093/infdis/jiz656.

10. Kim UJ, Won EJ, Kee SJ, et al. Combination therapy with lopinavir/ritonavir, ribavirin and interferon-alpha for Middle East respiratory syndrome. Antivir Ther 2016;21(5):455–59.

11. Omrani AS, Saad MM, Baig K, et al. Ribavirin and interferon alfa-2a for severe Middle East respiratory syndrome coronavirus infection: A retrospective cohort study. Lancet Infect Dis 2014;14(11):1090–95.

12. Chu CM, Cheng VC, Hung IF, et al. Role of lopinavir/ritonavir in the treatment of SARS: initial virological and clinical fndings. Thorax 2004;59(3):252–56.

13. Cao B, Wang Y, Wen D, et al. A Trial of lopinavir-ritonavir in adults hospitalized with severe COVID-19. N Engl J Med 2020. https://doi.org/10.1056/ NEJMoa2001282

14. Mulangu S, Dodd LE, Davey RT Jr, et al. A randomized, controlled trial of ebola virus disease therapeutics. N Engl J Med 2019;381(24):2293–303.

15. Gordon CJ, Tchesnokov EP, Feng JY, et al. The antiviral compound remdesivir potently inhibits RNA-dependent RNA polymerase from Middle East respiratory syndrome coronavirus. J Biol Chem 2020. https://doi. org/10.1074/jbc.AC120.013056.

16. de Wit E, Feldmann F, Cronin J, et al. Prophylactic and therapeutic remdesivir (GS-5734) treatment in the rhesus macaque model of MERSCoV infection. Proc Natl Acad Sci USA 2020. https://doi.org/10.1073/ pnas.1922083117.

17. Sheahan TP, Sims AC, Leist SR, et al. Comparative therapeutic efcacy of remdesivir and combination lopinavir, ritonavir, and interferon beta against MERS-CoV. Nat Communs 2020;11(1):222.

18. Holshue ML, DeBolt C, Lindquist S, et al. First case of 2019 novel coronavirus in the United States. N Engl J Med 2020;382(10):929–36.

19. Blaising J, Polyak SJ, Pecheur EI. Arbidol as a broad-spectrum antiviral: an update. Antiviral Res 2014;107:84–94.

20. Boriskin YS, Leneva IA, Pecheur EI, et al. Arbidol: A broad-spectrum antiviral compound that blocks viral fusion. Curr Med Chem. 2008;15(10):997–1005.

21. Khamitov RA, Loginova S, Shchukina VN, et al. Antiviral activity of arbidol and its derivatives against the pathogen of severe acute respiratory syndrome in the cell cultures. Vopr Virusol 2008;53(4):9–13.

22. Lu H. Drug treatment options for the 2019-new coronavirus (2019-nCoV). Biosci Trends 2020. https://doi.org/10.5582/bst.2020.01020.

23. Qu J. Clinical study of arbidol hydrochloride tablets in the treatment of pneumonia caused by novel coronavirus, 2020. https://clinicaltrials.gov/ ct2/show/NCT04260594. Accessed 7 Feb 2020.

24. Li W, Moore MJ, Vasilieva N, et al. Angiotensin-converting enzyme 2 is a functional receptor for the SARS coronavirus. Nature 2003;426(6965):450–54.

25. Dimitrov DS. The secret life of ACE2 as a receptor for the SARS virus. Cell 2003;115(6): 652–53.

26. Simmons G, Reeves JD, Rennekamp AJ, et al. Characterization of severe acute respiratory syndrome-associated coronavirus (SARS-CoV) spike glycoprotein-mediated viral entry. Proc Natl Acad Sci USA 2004;101(12):4240–45.

27. Yeung KS, Yamanaka GA, Meanwell NA. Severe acute respiratory syndrome coronavirus entry into host cells: Opportunities for therapeutic intervention. Med Res Rev 2006;26(4):414–33.

28. Yan Y, Zou Z, Sun Y, et al. Anti-malaria drug chloroquine is highly efective in treating avian infuenza A H5N1 virus infection in an animal model. Cell Res 2013;23(2):300–02.

29. Vincent MJ, Bergeron E, Benjannet S, et al. Chloroquine is a potent inhibitor of SARS coronavirus infection and spread. Virol J 2005;2:69.

30. Xu H, Zhong L, Deng J, et al. High expression of ACE2 receptor of 2019-nCoV on the epithelial cells of oral mucosa. Int J Oral Sci 2020;12(1):8.

31. Wang M, Cao R, Zhang L, et al. Remdesivir and chloroquine efectively inhibit the recently emerged novel coronavirus (2019-nCoV) in vitro. Cell Res 2020. https://doi.org/10.1038/ s41422-020-0282-0

32. Gao J, Tian Z, Yang X. Breakthrough: Chloroquine phosphate has shown apparent efficacy in treatment of COVID-19 associated pneumonia in clinical studies. Biosci Trends 2020;14(1):72–73.

33. Ponticelli C, Moroni G. Hydroxychloroquine in systemic lupus erythematosus (SLE). Expert Opin Drug Saf 2017;16(3):411–19.

34. Schrezenmeier E, Dorner T. Mechanisms of action of hydroxychloroquine and chloroquine: implications for rheumatology. Nat Rev Rheumatol 2020;16(3):155–66.

35. Yao X, Ye F, Zhang M, et al. In vitro antiviral activity and projection of optimized dosing design of hydroxychloroquine for the treatment of severe acute respiratory syndrome Coronavirus 2 (SARS-CoV-2). Clin Infect Dis 2020. https://doi.org/10.1093/cid/ciaa237.

36. Huang C, Wang Y, Li X, et al. Clinical features of patients infected with 2019 novel coronavirus in Wuhan, China. Lancet 2020;395(10223):497–506.

37. Beigel JH, Nam HH, Adams PL, et al. Advances in respiratory virus therapeutics—A meeting report from the 6th isirv Antiviral Group conference. Antiviral Res 2019;167:45–67.

38. Chen N, Zhou M, Dong X, et al. Epidemiological and clinical characteristics of 99 cases of 2019 novel coronavirus pneumonia in Wuhan, China: A descriptive study. Lancet 2020;395(10223):507–13.

39. Zhao Z, Zhang F, Xu M, et al. Description and clinical treatment of an early outbreak of severe acute respiratory syndrome (SARS) in Guangzhou, PR China. J Med Microbiol 2003;52(Pt 8):715–20.

40. Ho JC, Ooi GC, Mok TY, et al. High-dose pulse versus nonpulse corticosteroid regimens in severe acute respiratory syndrome. Am J Respir Crit Care Med 2003;168(12):1449–56.

41. Thompson BT. Glucocorticoids and acute lung injury. Crit Care Med 2003;31(4 Suppl): S253–57.

42. Ni YN, Chen G, Sun J, et al. The effect of corticosteroids on mortality of patients with infuenza pneumonia: a systematic review and meta-analysis. Crit Care 2019;23(1):99.

43. Yang JW, Fan LC, Miao XY, et al. Corticosteroids for the treatment of human infection with infuenza virus: A systematic review and metaanalysis. Clin Microbiol Infect 2015;21(10):956–63.

44. Martin-Loeches I, Lisboa T, Rhodes A, et al. Use of early corticosteroid therapy on ICU admission in patients afected by severe pandemic (H1N1)v infuenza A infection. Intensive Care Med 2011;37(2):272–83.

45. Arabi YM, Mandourah Y, Al-Hameed F, et al. Corticosteroid therapy for critically Ill patients with Middle East respiratory syndrome. Am J Respir Crit Care Med 2018;197(6):757–67.

46. Han K, Ma H, An X, et al. Early use of glucocorticoids was a risk factor for critical disease and death from pH1N1 infection. Clin Infect Dis 2011;53(4):326–33.

47. Bouadma L, Lescure FX, Lucet JC, Yazdanpanah Y, Timsit JF. Severe SARS-CoV2 infections: Practical considerations and management strategy for intensivists. Intensive Care Med 2020. https://doi.org/10.1007/s00134-020-05967-x

48. Brunkhorst FM, Weigand MA, Pletz M, Gastmeier P, Lemmen SW, Meier-Hellmann A, et al. S3 guideline sepsis-prevention, diagnosis, treatment, and aftercare: Summary of the strong recommendations. Med Klin Intensivmed Notfmed 2020;115(3):178–88. https://doi.org/10.1007/s00063-020-00671-6

49. Chen C, Zhang XR, Ju ZY, et al. Advances in the research of cytokine storm mechanism induced by Corona Virus Disease 2019 and the corresponding immunotherapies. Zhonghua Shao Shang Za Zhi 2020;36:E005.

50. Hofman E, Rahat MA, Feld J, et al. Efects of tocilizumab, an anti-interleukin-6 receptor antibody, on serum lipid and Adipokine levels in patients with rheumatoid arthritis. Int J Mol Sci 2019;20:18.

51. Le RQ, Li L, Yuan W, et al. FDA approval summary: tocilizumab for treatment of chimeric antigen receptor T cell-induced severe or life-threatening cytokine release syndrome. Oncologist 2018;23(8):943–47.

52. Diagnosis and Treatment Protocol for Novel Coronavirus Pneumonia (Trial Version 7). National Health Commission & State Administration of Traditional Chinese Medicine. 2020. http://healthcareus.sakura.ne.jp/wordp ress/2020/03/17/diagnosis-and-treatment-protocol-for-novel-coronaviru s-pneumonia-trial-version-7/. Accessed 17 Mar 2020.

53. Pfeferle S, Schopf J, Kogl M, et al. The SARS-coronavirus-host interactome: identifcation of cyclophilins as target for pan-coronavirus inhibitors. PLoS Pathog 2011;7(10):e1002331.

54. Matteucci C, Grelli S, Balestrieri E, et al. Thymosin alpha 1 and HIV-1: Recent advances and future perspectives. Fut Microbiol 2017;12:141–55.

55. Pica F, Gaziano R, Casalinuovo IA, et al. Serum thymosin alpha 1 levels in normal and pathological conditions. Expert Opin Biol Ther 2018;18(sup1):13–21.

56. Wu J, Zhou L, Liu J, et al. The efcacy of thymosin alpha 1 for severe sepsis (ETASS): a multicenter, single-blind, randomized and controlled trial. Crit Care 2013;17(1):R8.

57. Gao ZC, Zhu JH, Sun Y, et al. Clinical investigation of outbreak of nosocomial severe acute respiratory syndrome. Zhongguo Wei Zhong Bing Ji Jiu Yi Xue 2003;15(6):332–35

58. Morgenstern B, Michaelis M, Baer PC, et al. Ribavirin and interferon-beta synergistically inhibit SARS-associated coronavirus replication in animal and human cell lines. Biochem Biophys Res Commun 2005;326(4):905–08.

59. Mustafa S, Balkhy H, Gabere MN. Current treatment options and the role of peptides as potential therapeutic components for Middle East Respiratory Syndrome (MERS): A review. J Infect Public Health 2018;11(1):9–17.

60. Kuri T, Zhang X, Habjan M, et al. Interferon priming enables cells to partially overturn the SARS coronavirus-induced block in innate immune activation. J Gen Virol 2009;90(Pt 11):2686–94.

61. Werdan K, Pilz G, Bujdoso O, et al. Score-based immunoglobulin G therapy of patients with sepsis: the SBITS study. Crit Care Med 2007;35(12):2693–2701.

62. Alejandria MM, Lansang MA, Dans LF, et al. Intravenous immunoglobulin for treating sepsis, severe sepsis and septic shock. Cochrane Database Syst Rev 2013. https://doi.org/10.1002/14651858.CD001090. pub2(9):Cd001090.

63. Marano G, Vaglio S, Pupella S, et al. Convalescent plasma: new evidence for an old therapeutic tool? Blood Trans 2016;14(2):1–6.

64. Burnouf T, Conton B, Dye JM. Convalescent plasma for Ebola virus disease. N Engl J Med 2016;374(25):2498–500.

65. Soo YO, Cheng Y, Wong R, et al. Retrospective comparison of convalescent plasma with continuing high-dose methylprednisolone treatment in SARS patients. Clin Microbiol Infect 2004;10(7):676–78.

66. Cheng Y, Wong R, Soo YO, et al. Use of convalescent plasma therapy in SARS patients in Hong Kong. Eur J Clin Microbiol Infect Dis 2005;24(1):44–6.

67. Lu CL, Murakowski DK, Bournazos S, et al. Enhanced clearance of HIV1-infected cells by broadly neutralizing antibodies against HIV-1 in vivo. Science 2016;352(6288):1001–04.

68. Zhao J, Perera RA, Kayali G, et al. Passive immunotherapy with dromedary immune serum in an experimental animal model for Middle East respiratory syndrome coronavirus infection. J Virol 2015;89(11):6117–20.

69. Uyeki TM, Bernstein HH, Bradley JS, et al. clinical practice guidelines by the infectious diseases society of America: 2018 update on diagnosis, treatment, chemoprophylaxis, and institutional outbreak management of seasonal infuenza. Clin Infect Dis 2019;68(6):895–902.

70. Wang D, Hu B, Hu C, Zhu F, Liu X, Zhang J, Wang B, Xiang H, Cheng Z, Xiong Y, Zhao Y, Li Y, Wang X, Peng Z. Clinical characteristics of 138 hospitalized patients with 2019 novel coronavirus-infected pneumonia in Wuhan, China. JAMA 2020. doi: 10.1001/jama.2020.1585.

71. Fowler RA, Lapinsky SE, Hallett D, et al. Critically ill patients with severe acute respiratory syndrome. JAMA 2003;290(3):367–73.

72. Frat JP, Thille AW, Mercat A, et al. High-fow oxygen through nasal cannula in acute hypoxemic respiratory failure. N Engl J Med 2015;372(23):2185–96.

73. Hui DS, Chow BK, Lo T, et al. Exhaled air dispersion during high-fow nasal cannula therapy versus CPAP via diferent masks. Eur Respir J 2019;53:4.

74. Hui DS, Chow BK, Chu L, et al. Exhaled air dispersion during coughing with and without wearing a surgical or N95 mask. PLoS ONE 2012;7(12):e50845.

75. Society RccoCT. Expert consensus on preventing nosocomial transmission during respiratory care for critically ill patients infected by 2019 novel coronavirus pneumonia. Zhonghua Jie He He Hu Xi Za Zhi 2020;17:E020.

76. Kumar A, Zarychanski R, Pinto R, et al. Critically ill patients with 2009 infuenza A(H1N1) infection in Canada. JAMA 2009;302(17):1872–79.

77. Rochwerg B, Brochard L, Elliott MW, et al. Official ERS/ATS clinical practice guidelines: noninvasive ventilation for acute respiratory failure. Eur Respir J 2017;50:2.

78. Cheung JC, Ho LT, Cheng JV, Cham EYK, Lam KN. Staff safety during emergency airway management for COVID-19 in Hong Kong. Lancet Respir Med 2020. https://doi.org/10.1016/S2213–2600(20)30084–9.

79. Lewis SR, Butler AR, Parker J, Cook TM, Schofield-Robinson OJ, Smith AF. Videolaryngoscopy versus direct laryngoscopy for adult patients requiring tracheal intubation: A Cochrane Systematic Review. Br J Anaesth 2017;119: 369–83.

80. World Health Organization (2020, March 14) Clinical management of severe acute respiratory infection (SARI) when COVID-19 disease is suspected.

81. Slutsky AS, Ranieri VM. Ventilator-induced lung injury. N Engl J Med 2013; 369: 2126–36.

82. Alhazzani W, Moller MH, Arabi YM, et al. Surviving Sepsis Campaign: guidelines on the management of critically ill adults with Coronavirus Disease 2019 (COVID-19). Intensive Care Med 2020. https://doi.org/10.1007/s00134-020-06022-5.

83. Brower RG, Matthay MA, Morris A, Schoenfeld D, Thompson BT, Wheeler A, Acute Respiratory Distress Syndrome Network. Ventilation with lower tidal volumes as compared with traditional tidal volumes for acute lung injury and the acute respiratory distress syndrome. N Engl J Med 2000;342:1301–08.

84. Guerin C, Reignier J, Richard JC, Beuret P, Gacouin A, Boulain T, et al, PROSEVA Study Group. Prone positioning in severe acute respiratory distress syndrome. New England Journal of Medicine 2013 Jun 6;368(23):2159–68.

85. Reignier J, Dimet J, Martin-Lefevre L, Bontemps F, Fiancette M, Clementi E, et al. Before-after study of a standardized ICU protocol for early enteral feeding in patients turned in the prone position. Clinical Nutrition 2010 Apr;29(2):210–16.

86. Cornejo RA, Diaz JC, Tobar EA, Bruhn AR, Ramos CA, Gonzalez RA, Repetto CA, Romero CM, Galvez LR, Llanos O, Arellano DH, Neira WR, Diaz GA, Zamorano AJ, Pereira GL. Effects of prone positioning on lung protection in patients with acute respiratory distress syndrome. Am J Respir Crit Care Med 2013;188: 440–48.

87. Xu Y, Deng X, Han Y, et al. A multicenter retrospective review of prone position ventilation (PPV) in treatment of severe human H7N9 Avian flu. PLoS ONE 2015;10(8):e0136520.

88. Albert RK, Hubmayr RD. The prone position eliminates compression of the lungs by the heart. Am J Respir Crit Care Med 2000;161: 1660–65.

89. Nyren S, Radell P, Lindahl SG, Mure M, Petersson J, Larsson SA, Jacobsson H, Sanchez-Crespo A. Lung ventilation and perfusion in prone and supine postures with reference to anesthetized and mechanically ventilated healthy volunteers. Anesthesiology 2010;112: 682–87.

90. Hardin CC, Hibbert K. ECMO for severe acute respiratory distress syndrome. New England Journal of Medicine 2018 Sep 13;379(11):1092–93.

91. Noah MA, Peek GJ, Finney SJ, et al. Referral to an extracorporeal membrane oxygenation center and mortality among patients with severe 2009 infuenza A(H1N1). JAMA 2011;306(15):1659–68.

92. Alshahrani MS, Sindi A, Alshamsi F, et al. Extracorporeal membrane oxygenation for severe Middle East respiratory syndrome coronavirus. Ann Intensive Care 2018;8(1):3.

93. Wang D, Hu B, et al. Clinical characteristics of 138 hospitalized patients with 2019 novel coronavirus-infected pneumonia in Wuhan, China. JAMA 2020. https://doi.org/10.1001/jama.2020.1585.

94. MacLaren G, Fisher D, Brodie D. Preparing for the most critically ill patients with COVID-19: The potential role of extracorporeal membrane oxygenation. JAMA 2020. https://doi.org/10.1001/jama.2020.2342.

95. Bentzer P, Griesdale DE, Boyd J, MacLean K, Sirounis D, Ayas NT. Will this hemodynamically unstable patient respond to a bolus of intravenous fluids? JAMA 2016;316: 1298–1309.

96. Pan J, Peng M, Liao C, Hu X, Wang A, Li X. Relative efficacy and safety of early lactate clearance-guided therapy resuscitation in patients with sepsis: A meta-analysis. Medicine (Baltimore) 2019;98:e14453.

97. Hernandez G, Ospina-Tascon GA, Damiani LP, Estenssoro E, Dubin A, et al. Effect of a resuscitation strategy targeting peripheral perfusion status vs serum lactate levels on 28-day mortality among patients with septic shock: The ANDROMEDA-SHOCK Randomized Clinical Trial. JAMA 2019;321:654–64.

98. McClave SA, Taylor BE, Martindale RG, Warren MM, Johnson DR, Braunschweig C, et al. Society of Critical Care Medicine; American Society for Parenteral and Enteral Nutrition. Guidelines for the provision and assessment of nutrition support therapy in the adult critically ill patient: Society of Critical Care Medicine (SCCM) and American Society for Parenteral and Enteral Nutrition (ASPEN). JPEN J Parenter Enteral Nutr 2016 Feb;40(2):159–211.

99. Taylor BE, McClave SA, Martindale RG, Warren MM, Johnson DR, Braunschweig C, et al. Society of Critical Care Medicine; American Society of Parenteral and Enteral Nutrition. Guidelines for the provision and assessment of nutrition support therapy in the adult critically ill patient: Society of Critical Care Medicine (SCCM) and American Society for Parenteral and Enteral Nutrition (ASPEN). Critical Care Medicine. 2016 Feb;44(2):390–438.

100. Singer P, Blaser AR, Berger MM, Alhazzani W, Calder PC, Casaer MP, et al. ESPEN guideline on clinical nutrition in the intensive care unit. Clinical Nutrition 2019 Feb;38(1):48–79.

101. Patel JJ, Rice T, Heyland DK. Safety and outcomes of early enteral nutrition in circulatory shock. JPEN J Parenter Enteral Nutr 2020 Feb 12. doi: 10.1002/jpen.1793.

102. Arabi YM, McClave SA. Enteral nutrition should not be given to patients on vasopressor agents. Critical Care Medicine 2020 Jan;48(1):119–21.

103. Gu J, Han B, Wang J. COVID-19: Gastrointestinal manifestations and potential fecal-oral transmission. Gastroenterology 2020 Mar 3. doi: https://doi.org/10.1053/j.gastro.2020.02.054.

104. Pan L, Mu M, Yang P, Sun Y, et al. Clinical characteristics of COVID-19 patients with digestive symptoms in Hubei, China: a descriptive, cross-sectional, multicenter study. American Journal of Gastroenterology 2020 Mar 18. https://journals.lww.com/ajg/Documents/COVID_Digestive_Symptoms_AJG_Preproof.pdf

105. Xiao F, Tang M, Zheng X, et al. Evidence for gastrointestinal infection of SARS-CoV-2. Gastroenterology 2020 Mar 3. https://doi.org/10.1053/j.gastro.2020.02.055.

106. Reignier J, Boisramé-Helms J, Brisard L, Lascarrou JB, Ait Hssain A, Anguel N, et al. NUTRIREA-2 Trial Investigators; Clinical Research in Intensive Care and Sepsis (CRICS) group. Enteral versus parenteral early nutrition in ventilated adults with shock: A randomised, controlled, multicentre, open-label, parallel-group study (NUTRIREA-2). Lancet 2018 Jan 13;391(10116):133–43.

107. Mehta P, McAuley DF, Brown M, Sanchez E, Tattersall RS, Manson JJ, et al., HLH Across Speciality Collaboration, UK. COVID-19: Consider cytokine storm syndromes and immunosuppression. Lancet 2020 Mar 28;395(10229):1033–34.

108. Reignier J, Mercier E, Le Gouge A, Boulain T, Desachy A, Bellec F, et al. Clinical Research in Intensive Care and Sepsis (CRICS) Group. Effect of not monitoring residual gastric volume on risk of ventilator-associated pneumonia in adults receiving mechanical ventilation and early enteral feeding: a randomized controlled trial. JAMA 2013 Jan 16;309(3):249–56.

109. Saez de la Fuente I, Saez de la Fuente J, Quintana Estelles MD, Garcia Gigorro R, Terceros Almanza LJ, Sanchez Izguierdo JA, et al. Enteral nutrition in patients receiving mechanical ventilation in a prone position. JPEN J Parenter Enteral Nutr 2016 Feb;40(2):250–55.

110. van der Voort PH, Zandstra DF. Enteral feeding in the critically ill: comparison between the supine and prone positions: A prospective crossover study in mechanically ventilated patients. Crit Care 2001;5: 216–20.

111. Reintam Blaser A, Starkopf J, Alhazzani W, Berger MM, Casaer MP, Deane AM, Fruhwald S, Hiesmayr M, Ichai C, Jakob SM, Loudet CI, Malbrain ML, Montejo Gonzalez JC, Paugam-Burtz C, Poeze M, Preiser JC, Singer P, van Zanten AR, De Waele J, Wendon J, Wernerman J, Whitehouse T, Wilmer A, Oudemans-van Straaten HM, Function EWGoG . Early enteral nutrition in critically ill patients: ESICM clinical practice guidelines. Intensive Care Med 2017;43: 380–98.

112. Kallet RH. The vexing problem of ventilator-associated pneumonia: Observations on pathophysiology, public policy, and clinical science. Respiratory Care 2015 Oct;60(10):1495–1508.

113. Ridley EJ, Davies AR, Robins EJ, Lukas G, Bailey MJ, Fraser JF. Nutrition therapy in adult patients receiving extracorporeal membrane oxygenation: A prospective, multicentre, observational study. Critical Care and Resuscitation 2015 Sep;17(3):183–89.

114. Bear DE, Smith E, Barrett NA. Nutrition support in adult patients receiving extracorporeal membrane oxygenation. Nutr Clin Pract 2018 Dec;33(6):738–46.

115. Ohbe H, Jo T, Yamana H, Matsui H, Fushimi K, Yasunaga H. Early enteral nutrition for cardiogenic or obstructive shock requiring venoarterial extracorporeal membrane oxygenation: A nationwide inpatient database study. Intensive Care Medicine 2018 Aug;44(8):1258–65.

116. Center of Disease Control (2020, February 14) Interim Guidelines for Collecting, Handling, and Testing Clinical Specimens from Persons Under Investigation (PUIs) for Coronavirus Disease 2019 (COVID-19). In: Book Interim Guidelines for Collecting, Handling, and Testing Clinical Specimens from Persons Under Investigation (PUIs) for Coronavirus Disease 2019 (COVID-19). City, pp.

117. Linton NM, Kobayashi T, Yang Y, Hayashi K, Akhmetzhanov AR, Jung SM, Yuan B, Kinoshita R, Nishiura H. Incubation Period and Other Epidemiological Characteristics of 2019 Novel Coronavirus Infections with Right Truncation: A Statistical Analysis of Publicly Available Case Data. J Clin Med 2020.doi: 10.3390/jcm9020538.

118. Chan PK, To WK, Ng KC, Lam RK, Ng TK, Chan RC, Wu A, Yu WC, Lee N, Hui DS, Lai ST, Hon EK, Li CK, Sung JJ, Tam JS. Laboratory diagnosis of SARS. Emerg Infect Dis 2004;10: 825–31.

119. Wu X, Cai Y, Huang X, Yu X, Zhao L, Wang F, Li Q, Gu S, Xu T, Li Y, Lu B, Zhan Q. Co-infection with SARS-CoV-2 and Influenza A Virus in Patient with Pneumonia, China. Emerg Infect Dis 2020. doi: 10.3201/eid2606.200299.

COVID-19 in Pregnancy

Ruchi Birendra, Shikha Sachan, Anjali Rani

INTRODUCTION

We are living in an unprecedented time where the data regarding COVID-19 is still emerging and we have very little initial data to support our guidelines, so as the humankind battles this severe acute respiratory infection (SARI), available information and the guidelines are also changing. Pregnancy is known to alter the body's immune system and response to viral infections in general, this can be seen as more severe symptoms in pregnant women, as was seen in other related coronavirus infections (including severe acute respiratory syndrome coronavirus (SARS-CoV). It was postulated based on this that pregnant women might have severe symptoms, morbidity and mortality from COVID-19 than general population. But the reports emerging have shown no severe course of illness in pregnant women and hence Centers for Disease Control and Prevention (CDC) recently removed pregnant people from their webpage that outlines "people who are at higher risk for severe illness" from COVID-19. The outcome of the disease is likely to be more adverse in patients with other comorbidities.

Most of the studies include major proportion of women in their third trimester, and as other coronavirus infections are known to cause first and second trimester complications like abortion, congenital malformations, foetal growth restriction (FGR), but enough data is not available to suggest whether the coronavirus can cause first and second trimester complications although high fever which is a hallmark of COVID infection, in first trimester can cause birth defects. Most of the preterm deliveries associated with COVID infection are supposed to be because doctors decided to risk a premature delivery because the moms-to-be were unwell. The data to show association of preterm delivery with COVID 19 is yet to be validated.

PREVENTION

Since the virus is transmitted from person to person by droplets, social distancing remains the key for reducing the risk of infection.

- To avoid contact with anyone suspected and showing symptoms of COVID-19.
- To avoid crowded public transport, if possible.
- If working professional, try and manage the work from home.

- To avoid large and small congregations even with family and friends and especially in closed or confined spaces.
- Use teleconsultation to contact your obstetrician, if unable to go for check-up.
- To regularly wash hands with water and soap. Use hand sanitizer with 60 to 95% alcohol.
- Stand 2 meters away from people, if the need arises to go outside, and avoid unnecessarily touching your nose and mouth.
- Take good nutrition and rest. Light exercises can be done after consultation with your doctor. Stay positive.

ANTENATAL CARE (ANC) VISITS

1. Since ANC is an essential care, it cannot be deferred for long. Avoiding antenatal care has been associated with increased event of adverse pregnancy outcomes for mother and fetus. Telecommunication can be done for minor ailments to prevent unnecessary hospital visits and also to plan for next visit. Routine ANC visits at 12, 20, 28 and 36 weeks is advised, if patient is not under self-isolation. Foetal kick count to be maintained.
2. All ANC patients should be triaged based on history and clinical presentation at the entrance of health facility into infected or potentially infected or clean cases. Infrared thermometer should be available with triage staff for screening.
3. If a woman meets criteria for COVID-19 testing, she should be tested. Until test results are available, she should be treated as though she has confirmed COVID-19.
4. For symptomatic patients, appointment should be postponed till 7 days after the start of symptom unless patient deteriorates.
5. Appointment should be deferred for 14 days for patients who are self-isolating due to exposure to COVID positive patient.
6. No additional tests are necessary, although growth scans are advisable, if patient was positive and required admission. Although studies are not yet available on association between FGR and COVID-19 infection, still growth scan is recommended 14 days after resolution of infection as there is association between FGR and SARS infection.
7. If ANC visits cannot be delayed until isolation period subsides, IPC practice is to be followed.
8. Obstetric intervention, if needed, should not be deferred awaiting COVID-19 result.
9. Suspected or confirmed COVID cases should use private transport or call 108 to reach the health facility. She should inform any maternity staff of her status before entering hospital. Woman should be attended by staff wearing PPE and taken to the isolation room designated for this purpose. Unnecessary staff and relatives should not be allowed to enter this room. Till the test results are available, the woman is to be treated as a confirmed case and infection prevention and control (IPC) to be followed strictly.
10. If routine appointment of woman is delayed for more than 3 weeks, she should contact ANMs/ASHAs in rural area by telephone or routine household visits with PPE.

11. Individualized plans for women requiring frequent review may be necessary. Women with additional comorbidities like diabetes, heart disease, bronchial asthma, immunosuppression require additional care as morbidity and mortality is considered to be high in this group of patients.

12. Women who are pregnant and are healthcare workers or partner of healthcare workers should take proper precaution of not coming in contact of positive or suspected positive cases.

13. MTP and abortion services being an essential healthcare should be continued to be provided.

CLINICAL PRESENTATION

Most pregnant women present with mild to moderate flu-like symptoms of cough, sore throat, and fever. A few may present with difficulty in breathing. Pregnant women with other comorbidities like diabetes, asthma may present with pneumonia and marked hypoxia. Immunocompromised and elderly pregnant women may present with atypical features such as fatigue, malaise, body ache and/or gastrointestinal symptoms like nausea and diarrhoea. Reported cases of COVID-19 pneumonia in pregnancy are milder and with good recovery.

MANAGEMENT OF COVID-19 INFECTION IN PREGNANCY

For all pregnant women, obtain a detailed travel history or whether she is coming from hot spot area or history of exposure to people with symptoms of COVID-19 or look for symptoms of COVID-19. ICMR recommends testing in case of travel history in last 14 days (6 March, 2020 onwards) or is a close contact of a laboratory proven positive patient or she is a healthcare worker herself or is hospitalized with features of severe acute respiratory illness. Pregnant women residing in containment area or in large migration gatherings/evacuees centre from hotspot districts presenting in labour or likely to deliver in next 5 days should be tested, even if asymptomatic. Some states are now recommending screening for every antenatal patient who visits hospital.

There should be a triage area at the entrance of health facility for screening of patients. Health facility should consider for a separate registration desk with physical barrier (glass or plastic screens) for patients coming with respiratory symptoms to minimize the contact between the health professional and patient. CDC recommends that a standardized questionnaire should be used to assess, if the patient meets the COVID-19 case definition. As we are in the middle of a pandemic, there should be a high level of suspicion for COVID-19.

Nasopharyngeal swab is taken and sent for RT-PCR which is currently recommended by ICMR. Nucleic acid amplification test (NAAT) is the gold standard test but is expensive.

Asymptomatic patients are to be monitored at home till reports are awaited. If test is negative, the monitoring is stopped. If SARS-CoV-2 test is positive, they are to be isolated at home for 14 days.

All symptomatic patients are to be hospitalized for isolation and observation of progress of symptoms in isolated room prefer with negative pressure (IRNP). If SARS-

CoV-2 test is negative, patients are isolated at home for 14 days. If symptoms persist, retest is to be done. If SARS-CoV test is positive, then patient is to be managed in a tertiary care hospital where maternal and foetal surveillance can be done.

After admission, patients with mild symptoms should receive routine obstetrical care. These patients can be considered for discharge unless there is another medical or obstetrical concern. These patients are advised to do self-monitoring and report to emergency, if symptomatic deterioration. For patients with moderate symptoms, a detailed assessment of the patient including monitoring vitals, oxygen saturation assessment along with relevant blood investigations needs to be done. The laboratory findings that have been seen with COVID-19 infection are leucopenia, lympho-cytopenia, mild thrombocytopenia, mild elevation of liver enzymes and other acute infection markers. Chest X-ray and CT scan with abdominal shield protect the fetus from radiation exposure may be done, if needed. Patients with severe symptoms should be managed in ICU by team of experts.

COVID-19 infection is as such not an indication for termination of pregnancy or induction of labour. Decision regarding termination to be based on clinical judgement of the treating obstetrician but ICMR recommends to consider for cesarean delivery, if the patient is in septic shock or there are signs of acute organ failure or if there is foetal distress. If preterm delivery is anticipated, glucocorticoids can be given but there is no documented evidence of their use in COVID infection. However, their use needs to be individualized as glucocorticoids were associated with increased risk for mortality in patients with influenza and delayed viral clearance in patients.

Symptomatic treatment of patient is done with IV fluid, oxygen, and antipyretics. (Paracetamol is preferred and other NSAIDs may be avoided because there are concerns about potentiating ACE receptors.)

Hydroxychloroquine to be given 400 mg twice a day on day 1 and then 400 mg once a day for the next 4 days. Chloroquine at the dose of 500 mg twice a day for 7 days is another alternative.

VERTICAL TRANSMISSION

With regard to vertical transmission (transmission from mother to baby antenatally or intrapartum), emerging evidence now suggests that vertical transmission is probable, although the number of pregnancies affected and the number known to us and its significance to the newborn has yet to be determined. Previous case reports from China suggested little evidence for vertical transmission and no evidence that virus is transmitted in the amniotic fluid, cord blood. Virus was also found to be absent in swabs taken from neonate throat, placenta, genital fluid of mother.[1] A new report published on Thursday 26 March 2020 describes a single maternal–neonatal pair in which the infant born to a COVID-19 positive mother was found to have SARS-COV-2 IgM in serum at birth. Since IgM does not cross the placenta, this is likely to represent a neonatal immune response to *in utero* infection. ICMR has given in its guideline that vertical transmission is probable although its significance in causing the disease in newborn is not known.[2]

MODE AND PLACE OF DELIVERY

All deliveries should be attended at medical institution.[3,4] Uncomplicated deliveries could be handled at primary health centres but mode of termination should be at hand, if there arises a complication. High-risk deliveries could be handled at a tertiary care centre with NICU facilities. There should be a separate dedicated COVID labour room and operation theatre for positive and suspected patients, where proper precautions are taken by healthcare providers. This measure helps in keeping healthcare workers and another pregnant patient safe.

There should be written SOP (standard operating procedure) for labour room management for COVID-infected women.

As soon as the patient reports to labour room, she should be received by staff who has properly donned PPE. Reporting of COVID-19 patient should be done. Triage should be done and then decision should be taken for admission in labour room. Indications for admission in labour room remains same for COVID patients as for other obstetric patients. Delivery in birthing pool should not be allowed for COVID patients. Assessment of severity of symptoms should be done and patient should be managed as mentioned previously in the chapter.

Confirmation of the onset of labour is done as per standard care. Maternal observation is done by monitoring temperature, respiratory rate and oxygen saturation which should be >94%. Electronic foetal monitoring using cardiotocograph (CTG) is recommended in labour.

Only one birth attendant can be allowed. Minimum staff should be allowed. Patient should be given psychological support to reduce stress, fear and depression.

Neonatal resuscitation corner should be at least 2 meters away from the delivery table.

Intrapartum services should be provided in a way that minimum staff is engaged, with reference to requirements and the ability to provide emergency obstetric, anaesthetic and neonatal care where indicated.

If the patient develops hypoxia during intrapartum period, then forceps or vacuum can be used to cut short the 2nd stage of labour.

Only obstetric indications will decide whether the women will deliver vaginally or by caesarian section, however, there are some concerns regarding performing a caesarean section in active case might cause worsening of patient condition.

Donning of PPE must be done by the health professionals. But it is must even, if it delays the time of delivery of baby. Normally obstetricians in case of emergency do not take care of themselves. There are limited doctors for large population and they should take all precautions for the welfare of large population.

Evidences against the use of regional or spinal analgesia or anaesthesia is not present so it can be used in patients where urgent delivery is needed to minimize the use of general anaesthesia.

It should be kept in mind that intubating a patient for giving general anaesthesia for caesarean section is an aerosol generating procedure and should be performed by the team after taking due precautions.

Cleaning of operation theatre and equipment is very important. It can be done with 1% sodium hypochlorite solution.

Care should be taken while transporting the patient from labour room to operation theatre and to isolation ward. The personnel involved in transporting should be properly trained and use PPE.

CRITICAL CARE MANAGEMENT IN ICU[5]

If the pregnant patient with COVID infection is critically ill, she should be managed in ICU by team of experts. She may require ventilatory support. There should be a separate ICU for COVID patients.

Pregnant women with any of the following features need ICU admission

- Respiratory rate >30 breaths/min
- Oxygen saturation <93% at a rest
- Arterial partial pressure of oxygen (PaO_2)/oxygen concentration (FiO_2) <300 mmHg
- Patients with >50% lesions progression within 24 to 48 hours in lung imaging.
- Quick sequential organ failure assessment (qSOFA) score can be a useful adjunct to decision making for ICU. It includes 1 point for each of 3 criteria. qSOFA score ≥2 is suggestive of sepsis and needs intensive care. It includes following three points:
  1. Respiratory rate ≥22 breaths/min—1 point
  2. Mental status altered—1 point
  3. Systolic blood pressure ≤100 mmHg—1 point

BREASTFEEDING

There is no evidence to show that the virus is transmitted through breast milk, however, there are certain precautions that a suspected or COVID positive patient can take, if she decides to feed the baby after proper consultation with the healthcare provider.

While feeding the baby

- She should wear a face mask.
- Wash her hands thoroughly before touching her baby; be sure to get under your nails and into the webbing of your fingers.
- Wash her hands thoroughly before handling a breast pump or bottle.
- Considering having someone who is well give the baby a bottle of expressed breast milk.

Last option effectively minimizes the possibility of transmitting infection from mother to the neonate. If the mother is separated from the newborn, psychological support and counselling to the mother is to be provided.

Isolation, fear, financial difficulties, insecurity and inability to access support systems are all widely recognized risk factors for mental ill-health. The coronavirus epidemic increases the risk of perinatal anxiety and depression, as well as domestic violence. It is critically important that support for women and families is strengthened through the healthcare network as far as possible.

REFERENCES

1. Chen H, Guo J, Wang C, et al. Clinical characteristics and intrauterine vertical transmission potential of COVID-19 infection in nine pregnant women: A retrospective review of medical records. Lancet 2020 doi: https://doi.org/10.1016/S0140-6736(20)30360-3
2. https://icmr.nic.in/sites/default/files/upload_documents/Guidance_for_Management_of_Pregnant_Women_in_COVID19_Pandemic_12042020.pdf visited on 22.04.20
3. RCOG guidelines: Coronavirus (COVID-19) Infection in Pregnancy, Information for healthcare professionals Version 5: Published Saturday 28 March 2020.
4. FOGSI GCPR guidelines: Pregnancy with COVID-19 Infection.
5. Centers for Disease Control and Prevention guidelines.

Paediatric Care

Abhishek Abhinay, SK Rao

AETIOLOGY

Coronavirus disease 2019 is an infection caused by the severe acute respiratory syndrome coronavirus 2 (SARS-CoV-2), which mainly affects the respiratory tract. The virus can also affect other organs such as the kidneys, heart, intestines, blood and nervous system. The disease has spread globally since identification of the first case in December 2019. The World Health Organization (WHO) named the illness as coronavirus disease 2019 (COVID-19) and declared it as a public health emergency and later a pandemic. The disease is contagious with human-to-human transmission via droplets from coughing, sneezing or direct contact. Transmission through faeces has also been reported. While COVID-19 has an incubation period of 14 (usually 3–7) days, infection may be transmitted even during this period.

EPIDEMIOLOGY

The impact of the disease due to the novel coronavirus, SARS-CoV-2, COVID-19 has been widespread, with 213 countries and territories around the world reporting a total of 94,35,610 cases with 4,81,968 deaths.[1] Children have accounted for 1–5% of diagnosed patients and are less likely to become severely ill or die as compared to adults.[2] In a series from China, 13% virologically confirmed patients had asymptomatic infection. Only 5% symptomatic children had dyspnoea or hypoxaemia, and 0.6% progressed to ARDS or multiorgan dysfunction.[3] While the severity of illness in children is less as compared to adults and preschool children whereas infants have severe illness. In India, the total number of cases on 24 June 2020 was 4,72,972 with 14,907 deaths.[4] Of confirmed cases, 80 were children with one death.[5] Cases of COVID-19 in India are presently related to travel and local transmission from imported cases to their contacts and from hotspots. In adults, the risk factors for mortality are older age and presence of co-morbidities like hypertension, cardiovascular diseases, diabetes, chronic respiratory diseases, and malignancy.[6]

CLINICAL MANIFESTATION

COVID-19 infections in paediatric age groups is relatively mild and have a better prognosis. Clinical features of COVID-19 in children include fever, dry cough and difficulty in breathing; similar to flu, other symptoms include expectoration, headache, haemoptysis and diarrhoea. Most of the infected children are asymptomatic and act as a carrier for transmission of the disease. In some patients, the disease can progress to pneumonia, respiratory failure and even death due to rapid rise in inflammatory cytokines including IL-2, IL-7, IL-10, G-CSF, IP-10, MCP-1, MIP-1A, and TNF-α secondary to host immune response.[7,8]

Children and young adults are less severely affected than older individuals this might be due to differential involvement of immune system function in the elderly and/or differences in the expression of the cellular receptor for SARS-CoV-2 angiotensin-converting enzyme 2.[9,10] Other suggested reasons include children having a more active innate immune response, healthier respiratory tracts because they have not been exposed to as much smoke and air pollution as compared to adults and have fewer underlying disorders.

LABORATORY STUDIES

Blood investigations are usually non-specific. The white blood cell count is typically normal or reduced with decreased neutrophil[11] and lymphopenia; a lymphocyte count <1000 has been associated with severe disease. ESR and C-reactive protein may be raised but procalcitonin levels are often normal and raised in concomitant bacterial infection. In severe cases, elevated liver enzymes, lactate dehydrogenase levels, as well as abnormal coagulation, thrombocytopenia and elevated D-dimers have been reported.[12–16]

RADIOLOGICAL IMAGING

The chest X-ray (CXR) usually shows bilateral infiltrates but may be normal in early disease. The CT is more sensitive and specific. CT imaging generally shows infiltrates, unilateral or bilateral subpleural ground glass opacities and subsegmental consolidation with surrounding halo sign. It is also abnormal in asymptomatic patients/patients with no clinical evidence of lower respiratory tract involvement. In fact, abnormal CT scans have been used to diagnose COVID-19 in suspect cases with negative molecular diagnosis; many of these patients had positive molecular tests on repeat testing.[17]

Moreover, since most of the paediatric patients are mild cases, plain chest X-ray often fails to show the lesions or the detailed features, leading to misdiagnosis or missed diagnosis. Therefore, early chest CT examination is useful. In some suspected paediatric patients with a negative nucleic acid of COVID-19 virus, management based on the typical lesions shown on chest CT, which could provide evidence not only for early treatment to the children but also for effectively isolating the source of infection.[18] The observation of lesions on chest CT lagged behind clinical symptoms and nucleic acid detection. Lesions could be still visible on chest CT when two consecutive nucleic acid tests were negative.

DIAGNOSIS

A clinically suspect case is defined as one with fever, sore throat and cough who has history of travel to China or other areas of persistent local transmission or contact with patients with similar travel history or those with confirmed COVID-19 infection.

However, cases may be asymptomatic or even without fever. A confirmed case is a suspect case with a positive molecular test.

In a clinical setting, COVID-19 has mostly been diagnosed using nasal or pharyngeal swabs or sputum specimens that were positive for 2019-nCoV nucleic acid using real-time, reverse transcriptase-polymerase chain reaction assays. However, due to the limitation of invasive specimen collection in paediatric cases, especially in the early stage of the disease, the positive rate is relatively low. Therefore, early diagnosis in clinically suspected cases with evident radiological finding may helpful during early course of treatment. Virus may also be detected in the stool and in severe cases in blood. Alternative diagnostics have included genetic sequencing of specimens from the respiratory tract or blood consistent with SARS-CoV-2. Serology has been used to diagnose infections with SARS-CoV, but is not useful in the acute phase of the infection.[19–22] Cross-reactivities between antibodies against SARS-CoV and common CoVs have been observed.[23] WHO does not currently recommend the use of antigen-detecting rapid diagnostic and antibody-detecting rapid diagnostic tests for patient care but encourages the continuation of work to establish their usefulness in disease surveillance and epidemiologic research.

DIFFERENTIAL DIAGNOSIS

Most of the viral infections causing respiratory illness having similar non-specific self-limiting symptoms, but may progress to severe disease.[24,25] The differential diagnosis includes all types of respiratory viral infections clinically manifested as flulike or lower respiratory tract symptoms [influenza, parainfluenza, respiratory syncytial virus (RSV), adenovirus, human metapneumovirus (hMPV) non-COVID-19 coronavirus], atypical organisms (*Mycoplasma, Chlamydia*) and bacterial infections. Among these, the most relevant is influenza, usually characterized by fever, myalgia, headache and non-productive cough that may also cause complications with high morbidity and mortality rate, such as pneumonia, myocarditis, central nervous system disease and death.[26, 27] Clinically and by routine tests, these infections are very difficult to differentiate. Therefore, travel history becomes important, however, in community spread during pandemic, the travel history will become insignificant.

TREATMENT
Treatment is essentially supportive and symptomatic.

Asymptomatic patients do not require any treatment and hospitalisation.

Mild symptomatic groups include fever, cough, cold, malaise without respiratory distress, feeding well and normal oxygen saturation at room air. This group of patients require supportive and symptomatic treatments. Antipyretic for fever, plenty of fluid and adequate calorie intake are required and not need to be hospitalized and require home isolation. Counselling of patients must be done regarding signs and symptoms of severity of the disease before sending home and specially explained them, when they to seek urgent care at health facilities during the period of isolation.

Severe symptomatic groups include features of mild illness plus signs of respiratory distress [fast breathing as per age cut off, cyanosis (SpO_2 <90%), severe retraction, lethargy, seizure]. All subset of patients presenting with severe symptoms should be hospitalized and provided specialized care as per need. Hypoxic patients require oxygen therapy either through nasal prongs; face mask, high flow nasal cannula (HFNC) or non-invasive ventilation, mechanical ventilation and even extracorporeal membrane oxygen support, if indicated. Dialysis may be required in case of renal derangements. If bacterial infection is suspected, give broad-spectrum antibiotics empirically to treat all likely pathogens causing SARI and sepsis as soon as possible, and then therapy should be shifted on the basis of microbiology results and condition of patients. Antifungal required, if co-infections are suspected or proven. Role of corticosteroids with nebulized interferon alpha 2b and oral lopinavir/ritonavir for complications like ARDS, encephalitis, hemophagocytic syndrome or septic shock has been not established and require well-designed studies to proof benefits in near future.[28] WHO does not advocate use of corticosteroids in COVID-19 ARDS, although preliminary observations from China suggest short-term therapy of steroids in COVID-19 ARDS.[29,30] The probable mechanism behind use of steroids may be because of their anti-inflammatory actions and to suppress host-mediated cytokines storm. Neither the World Health Organization (WHO) nor the US Centers for Disease Control and Prevention (CDC) recommends any specific treatment in children or adults.[31,32] However, prior studies showed[33] combination of hydroxychloroquine and azithromycin reduces viral loads as compared to routine care in adults. Therefore, we suggest hydroxychloroquine (7–8 mg/kg/dose twice daily for day 1 and then days 2–5, 7–8 mg/kg once a day), azithromycin (10 mg/kg/day for 5 to 7 days), zinc and vitamin C as per recommended daily allowance. Oseltamivir may be used in early course of treatment in dose of 30 mg BD if less than 15 kg weight, 45 mg BD, 60 mg BD, and 75 mg BD, in weight band of 16–23 kg, 24–40 kg and more than 40 kg, respectively. This drug should be stopped, if test report of H1N1 is negative.

SPECIFIC THERAPY

Currently the US Food and Drug Administration (FDA) has not approved any medications to treat patients with COVID-19 in paediatric age group. Results of multiple on-going clinical trials may become available in near future that will probably guide next line of treatment. Other drugs proposed for therapy are arbidol (an antiviral drug available in Russia and China), intravenous immunoglobulin, monoclonal antibodies, RNA synthesis inhibitor, chloroquine and plasma of patients recovered from COVID-19.[34–36]

PREVENTION

Community Level

At community level, people should try to avoid crowded areas and postpone non-essential travel to other places during transmission. Everyone should cover their nose and mouth with a tissue or elbow when coughing or sneezing (cough etiquettes)[37] and ensure hand hygiene. Hand cleansing can be done with soap and water or an alcohol-based hand rub, handwash is preferred, if hands are visibly soiled. Person with cough and cold should wear surgical masks. However, routine use of mask by healthy people in public places are advised because efficacy for prevention of acquisition of infections in masked condition. In unavoidable circumstances, physical distancing should be practiced.

Facility Level

Effective ways to prevent viral transmission especially in hospital settings are to minimize aerosol-generating procedures such as intubation and bronchoscopy. Nebulization and nasal continuous positive airway pressure systems should be avoided in open ward. If indicated, then use appropriate personal protective equipment (PPE— water resistant gowns, disposable gloves, N95 masks and goggles or face shields). Only suction catheters and mechanical respirators with a closed-circuit system and viral filters should be used. Hospital hygiene practices are, therefore, crucial to limit nosocomial outbreaks. Ideally, separate room should be allotted for each patient. If this is not possible, patients and healthcare workers should be cohorted.[38, 39] Distance between two patients' beds should be at least 1 meter and maintain social distancing regardless of whether they are suspected to have COVID-19. Visitors should be avoided or limited. Currently, no prophylaxis is recommended for children and should not be administered hydroxychloroquine.[40]

VACCINES

The main antigens for vaccine development are the structural spike glycoprotein S or its receptor-binding domain.[41] However, the propensity of CoVs to rapidly mutate and recombine poses a potential problem for vaccine development.[42–44] Furthermore, the enhanced disease after viral challenges post vaccination has been observed in animal models after several different vaccines.[45, 46] Other types of vaccines like, live-attenuated vaccines, inactivated vaccines, and subunit and recombinant vaccines, viral vectors vaccines and DNA vaccines are in under trial.

REFERENCES

1. World Health Organization. Coronavirus disease (COVID-19) Situation dashboard. Available: https://who.sprinklr.com/[Accessed 24 June 2020].
2. Ludvigsson JF. Systematic review of COVID-19 in children shows milder cases and a better prognosis than adults. Acta Paediatr 2020; Mar 23 [Epub ahead of print].
3. Dong Y, Mo X, Hu Y, Qi X, Jiang F, Jiang Z, Tong S. Epidemiology of COVID-19 Among Children in China. Pediatrics. 2020 Mar 16. [Epub ahead of print].
4. Ministry of Health and Family Welfare, Government of India. COVID-19 INDIA. Available: https://www.mohfw.gov.in/ [Accessed 24 June 2020].
5. India COVID-19 tracker. COVID19-India: Patient Database. Available: https://www.covid19india.org [Accessed 7 April 2020].
6. Wu C, Chen X, Cai Y, Xia J, Zhou X, Xu S, et al. Risk factors associated with acute respiratory distress syndrome and death in patients with coronavirus disease 2019 pneumonia in Wuhan, China. JAMA Intern Med 2020; Mar 13[Epub ahead of print].
7. Chen N, Zhou M, Dong X, et al. Epidemiological and clinical characteristics of 99 cases of 2019 novel coronavirus pneumonia in Wuhan, China: a descriptive study. Lancet. 2020; 395:507–13.
8. Kliegman RM, St Geme JW, Blum NJ, Shah SS, Takser RC, Wilson KM. Nelson Textbook of Pediatrics. Edition 20. Philadelphia, PA: Elsevier, 2020.
9. Lu R, Zhao X, Li J, Niu P, Yang B, Wu H, Wang W, et al. Genomic characterisation and epidemiology of 2019 novel coronavirus: implications for virus origins and receptor binding. Lancet 2020 doi: 10.1016/S0140-6736(20)30251–8.

10. Hofmann H, Pyrc K, van der Hoek L, Geier M, Berkhout B, Pöhlmann S. Human coronavirus NL63 employs the severe acute respiratory syndrome coronavirus receptor for cellular entry. Proc Natl Acad Sci USA 2005; 102: 7988–93.

11. Cheng FW, Ng PC, Chiu WK, et al. A case-control study of SARS versus community acquired pneumonia. Arch Dis Child. 2005; 90:747–9.

12. Hon KL, Leung CW, Cheng WT, et al. Clinical presentations and outcome of severe acute respiratory syndrome in children. Lancet. 2003; 361:1701–3.

13. Chiu WK, Cheung PC, Ng KL, et al. Severe acute respiratory syndrome in children: experience in a regional hospital in Hong Kong. Pediatr Crit Care Med. 2003; 4:279–83.

14. Bitnun A, Allen U, Heurter H, et al; Other Members of the Hospital for Sick Children SARS Investigation Team. Children hospitalized with severe acute respiratory syndrome-related illness in Toronto. Pediatrics. 2003;112: e261.

15. Chen ZM, Fu JF, Shu Q, et al. Diagnosis and treatment recommendations for pediatric respiratory infection caused by the 2019 novel coronavirus. World J Pediatr. 2020. [Epub ahead of print]

16. Leung CW, Kwan YW, Ko PW, et al. Severe acute respiratory syndrome among children. Pediatrics. 2004;113: e535–e543.

17. Huang P, Liu T, Huang L, etal. Use of chest CT in combination with negative RT-PCR assay for the 2019 novel coronavirus but high clinical suspicion. Radiology. 2020. https://doi.org/10.1148/radiol. 2020200330.

18. Xia W, Shao J, Guo Y, Peng X, Li Z, Hu D. Clinical and CT features in pediatric patients with COVID-19 infection: Different points from adults. Pediatric Pulmonology. 2020;1–6. https://doi.org/10.1002/ppul.24718.

19. Chen X, Zhou B, Li M, et al. Serology of severe acute respiratory syndrome: implications for surveillance and outcome. J Infect Dis. 2004; 189:1158–63.

20. Bermingham A, Heinen P, Iturriza-Gómara M, et al. Laboratory diagnosis of SARS. Philos Trans R Soc Lond B Biol Sci. 2004; 359:1083–9.

21. Zhao LQ, Qian Y, Zhu RN, et al. [Serological analysis of SARS coronavirus in children diagnosed clinically as severe acute respiratory syndrome cases during SARS epidemic in Beijing]. Zhonghua Er Ke Za Zhi. 2006; 44:262–6.

22. Müller MA, Meyer B, Corman VM, et al. Presence of Middle East respiratory syndrome coronavirus antibodies in Saudi Arabia: a nationwide, cross-sectional, serological study. Lancet Infect Dis. 2015; 15:559–64.

23. Che XY, Qiu LW, Liao ZY, et al. Antigenic cross-reactivity between severe acute respiratory syndrome-associated coronavirus and human coronaviruses 229E and OC43. J Infect Dis. 2005; 191:2033–7.

24. Follin P, Lindqvist A, Nyström K, Lindh M. A variety of respiratory viruses found in symptomatic travellers returning from countries with ongoing spread of the new influenza A(H1N1) v virus strain. Euro Surveill. 2009;14(24):19242. 10.2807/ese.14.24.19242-en [PubMed] [CrossRef] [Google Scholar].

25. Puro V, Minosse C, Cappiello G, Lauria FN, Capobianchi MR. Rhinovirus and lower respiratory tract infection in adults. Clin Infect Dis. 2005;40(7):1068-9. 10.1086/428359 [PubMed] [CrossRef] [Google Scholar].

26. Poehling KA, Edwards KM, Weinberg GA, Szilagyi P, Staat MA, Iwane MK, et al. The underrecognized burden of influenza in young children. N Engl J Med. 2006;355(1):31-40. 10.1056/NEJMoa054869 [PubMed] [CrossRef] [Google Scholar].

27. Centers for Disease Control and Prevention (CDC) Estimates of deaths associated with seasonal influenza, United States, 1976-2007. MMWR Morb Mortal Wkly Rep. 2010;59(33):1057-62. [PubMed] [Google Scholar].

28. Chen ZM, Fu JF, Shu Q, et al. Diagnosis and treatment recommendations for pediatric respiratory infection caused by the 2019 novel coronavirus. World J Pediatr. 2020. [Epub ahead of print].

29. Russell CD, Millar JE, Baillie JK. Clinical evidence does not support corticosteroid treatment for 2019-nCoV lung injury. Lancet. 2020; 395:473–5.

30. 3Zhao JP, Hu Y, Du RH, et al. Expert consensus on the use of corticosteroid in patients with 2019-nCoV pneumonia. Zhonghua Jie He Hu Xi Za Zhi. 2020;43: E007.

31. Czub M, Weingartl H, Czub S, et al. Evaluation of modified vaccinia virus Ankara based recombinant SARS vaccine in ferrets. Vaccine. 2005; 23:2273–9.

32. Centers for Disease Control and Prevention CfDCaP. Interim clinical guidance for management of patients with confirmed 2019 novel coronavirus (2019-nCoV) infection. 2020. Available at: https://www.cdc.gov/ coronavirus/2019-ncov/hcp/clinical-guidance-management-patients.html. Accessed February 21, 2010.

33. Morse JS, Lalonde T, Xu S, Liu WR. Learning from the past: possible urgent prevention and treatment options for severe acute respiratory infections caused by 2019-nCoV. Chembiochem. 2020; 21:730–8.

34. Jin YH, Cai L, Cheng ZS, et al. A rapid advice guideline for the diagnosis and treatment of 2019 novel coronavirus [2019-nCoV] infected pneumonia [standard version]. Mil Med Res. 2020; 7:4.

35. Zhang L, Liu Y. Potential interventions for novel coronavirus in China: a systemic review. J Med Virol. 2020. https://doi.org/10. 1002/jmv.25707.

36. Multicenter Collaboration Group of Department of Science and Technology of Guangdong Province and Health Commission of Guangdong Province for Chloroquine in the Treatment of Novel Coronavirus Pneumonia. [Expert consensus on chloroquine phosphate for the treatment of novel coronavirus pneumonia]. [Articlein Chinese] Zhonghua Jie He He Hu Xi Za Zhi. 2020;43: E019.

37. Singhal T. A Review of Coronavirus Disease-2019 (COVID-19). The Indian Journal of Pediatrics: https://doi.org/10.1007/s12098-020-03263-6.

38. Ng PC, So KW, Leung TF, et al. Infection control for SARS in a tertiary neonatal centre. Arch Dis Child Fetal Neonatal Ed. 2003;88: F405–F409.

39. Leung TF, Ng PC, Cheng FW, et al. Infection control for SARS in a tertiary pediatrics centre in Hong Kong. J Hosp Infect. 2004; 56:215–22.

40. Sankar J, Dhochak N, Kabra SK, Lodha R. COVID-19 in Children: Clinical Approach and Management. Indian J Pediatr. 2020;87(6):433-442. doi:10.1007/s12098-020-03292-1.

41. He Y, Li J, Du L, et al. Identification and characterization of novel neutralizing epitopes in the receptor-binding domain of SARS-CoV spike protein: revealing the critical antigenic determinants in inactivated SARS-CoV vaccine. Vaccine. 2006; 24:5498–5508.

42. Su S, Wong G, Shi W, et al. Epidemiology, genetic recombination, and pathogenesis of coronaviruses. Trends Microbiol. 2016; 24:490–502.

43. Kim DW, Kim YJ, Park SH, et al. Variations in spike glycoprotein gene of MERS-CoV, South Korea, 2015. Emerg Infect Dis. 2016; 22:100–4.

44. Sohrab SS, Azhar EI. Genetic diversity of MERS-CoV spike protein gene in Saudi Arabia. J Infect Public Health. 2019. [Epub ahead of print].

45. He Y, Zhou Y, Siddiqui P, et al. Inactivated SARS-CoV vaccine elicits high titers of spike protein-specific antibodies that block receptor binding and virus entry. Biochem Biophys Res Commun. 2004; 325:445–52.

46. Hashem AM, Algaissi A, Agrawal AS, et al. A highly immunogenic, protective, and safe adenovirus-based vaccine expressing Middle East respiratory syndrome coronavirus S1-CD40L fusion protein in a transgenic human dipeptidyl peptidase 4 mouse model. J Infect Dis. 2019; 220:1558–67.

Geriatric Care

Sankha Shubhra Chakrabarti, Upinder Kaur

INTRODUCTION

Severe acute respiratory syndrome coronavirus-2 (SARS-CoV-2) originated in all probability in China in late 2019 and spread worldwide over the next three to four months. The virus bears a 79% genetic similarity to the SARS-CoV which caused an epidemic in 2003, and shares stronger genetic similarity with bat and pangolin coronaviruses.[1] SARS-CoV-2 results in COVID-19 (coronavirus disease-2019) which is a predominantly respiratory syndrome but recently suggested to have more multisystem components, and has taken the form of a global pandemic with 94.35 lac confirmed cases and 4.81 lac deaths as on June 24th 2020.[2] The general trend worldwide has been an aggravated disease course and higher mortality and morbidity among elderly patients, especially those with chronic comorbidities.[3] This has raised questions on the effect of elderly immune changes on viral pathogenesis and its deleterious effects. It is also to be seen whether co-existing illnesses and polypharmacy which are prevalent in the elderly have some bearing on SARS-CoV-2 pathogenesis. Most nations in the world have responded to the COVID-19 challenge with a slew of health and administrative measures which include lockdowns. While these measures have been variably successful in tackling the pandemic, they have opened up new challenges for elderly patients, such as food security issues, accessibility of healthcare and psychiatric and care-provider issues. The elderly population in India is currently around 8.6% of the total population, with an age cutoff of 60 years being followed in India for geriatric practice. Although this is less than in developed countries, the absolute number of old people in India is huge and this is a vulnerable section of the population.[4] We intend to discuss the unique aspects of the SARS-CoV-2 pandemic with respect to the geriatric population.

COVID-19 IN THE ELDERLY—EPIDEMIOLOGICAL ASPECTS

Although COVID-19 has affected all races, ages and genders of the world population, an almost uniform finding has been excess morbidity and mortality in the elderly. A study from Wuhan, the epicenter of the epidemic reported a high percentage (70%) of severe or critical illness among the elderly.[5] In Italy, one of the European countries to be the earliest and worst hit by the pandemic, the case fatality rate (CFR) in those between 60 and 69 years, 70 and 79 years and ≥80 years were 3.5%, 12.8% and 20.2%, respectively whereas the CFR in all age group segments below 60 years were uniformly ≤1%. An important reason why Italy had a high absolute mortality was also the population demographic of the country. Italy has the second highest elderly population in the world after Japan (23% ≥65 years of age).[6] In addition, the availability of universal free healthcare in Italy, resulted in many elderly surviving till now to late ages, which would be impossible in other countries. Even among medical professionals with mortality in Italy, there is a disproportionately high number of elderly individuals. Indian data regarding pattern of mortality is still not available in the public domain but general clinical observations imply that severe COVID-19 illness in India too is affecting the elderly more. The pattern of deaths also seems to be similar to other nations.[3] In a way, India which has a lower percentage of people above 65 years of age, is naturally protected from COVID-related mortality. The implications of this would be clearer in the coming days.

IMMUNE CHANGES, CYTOKINE STORM AND COMORBIDITY IN ELDERLY AND IMPLICATIONS IN COVID-19

Immunosenescence

The phenomenon of immunosenescence is well-described in the elderly and refers to the gradual decline in immune function that occurs in individuals with aging. The changes that commonly occur include creation of a proinflammatory state, decrease in CD56+ NK cells, decreased mannose-binding lectins and complement system components, decline in the numbers of B cells, CD4+ cells, CD8+ cells and CD3+ cells, and a shift from Th1 to Th2 cytokine production.[7] The higher morbidity and mortality observed in elderly patients with COVID-19 may be a direct result of this decline in immune function, especially the decline in macrophage and granulocyte function and the age-related thymic involution—factors known to predispose to viral infections.[8] Likewise, the immune response to influenza vaccination in the elderly is poor. It has been observed that vaccination is effective in only 33% elderly persons in preventing clinical infection and in 74% in preventing mortality.[9] Thus, probable vaccine-induced immunity for SARS-CoV-2 may also be less likely in this population group. Most respiratory viral infections predispose the patient to secondary bacterial infections, especially in settings with poor hygiene practices. Often these superinfections are the main triggers of mortality in the patients. Immunosenescence may predispose the elderly to more secondary bacterial infections, thus causing an increase in mortality statistics.

Cytokine Storm

Enhanced and often dysregulated production of inflammatory cytokines (both pro- and anti-inflammatory) and chemokines; such as IL-1, IL-6, IL-10, TNFα, IL-17, etc. by immune effector cells in response to diverse pathologies is referred to as a cytokine storm. This has been described in the backdrop of several infections such as malaria, influenza, bacterial and fungal sepsis and most recently in COVID-19. It is thought to be the cause of multiple systemic and respiratory symptoms in COVID-19.[3,10–13] It is expected that due to the phenomenon of immunosenescence that takes place in the elderly, the cytokine storm may also have differential expression in the elderly. How this may impact morbidity and mortality as well as protection from COVID-19 in the elderly remains to be seen.

Comorbidity in Elderly

The maximum mortality and morbidity due to COVID-19 worldwide have been in patients with pre-existing comorbidities. In a study from New York city on 5700 patients hospitalized with COVID-19 (median age 63 years), hypertension, obesity and diabetes were present in 57%, 42% and 34% respectively, being the three commonest comorbidities.[14] A large study from China involving 1590 patients concluded that those with comorbidities had poorer outcomes in COVID-19 cases.[15] Early observations from news reports and government press releases in India also suggested a similar picture, while comprehensive studies are still lacking.[3] It is but natural that elderly patients would have a higher burden of comorbidities as well as would be on multidrug therapy for the same. This population is hence quite vulnerable to the complications of COVID-19.

DRUG INTERACTIONS AND PERSPECTIVES IN COVID-19 IN ELDERLY

At present, no antiviral is effective against SARS-CoV-2. Various trials are evaluating the efficacy of drugs such as ritonavir/lopinavir, remdesivir, chloroquine, interferon α, oseltamivir, faviprevir, macrolides and umifenovir. Clinical evidence on the use of these drugs is mentioned below.

- **Ritonavir/lopinavir:** These anti-HIV drugs have failed to produce significant clinical benefits in terms of time to clinical improvement in COVID-19 patients. Around 28% patients on ritonavir/lopinavir developed gastrointestinal disturbances.[16]

- **Remdesivir:** Like ritonavir/lopinavir, no considerable clinical benefits have been observed till date with remdesivir. 66% of patients on remdesivir developed adverse events, commoner being hypoalbuminaemia, liver derangements, constipation, and hypokalaemia.[17]

- **Chloroquine and hydroxychloroquine**: These antimalarial drugs have given good results in uncontrolled clinical studies. Evidence through RCTs is weak at present. They modulate the lysosomal pH and interfere with the activity of ACE2 receptor required for viral entry into the host cells. Such drugs should be given cautiously in elderly patients with underlying cardiovascular diseases because of the risk of ventricular tachycardia (VT), hypotension and bradycardia. Caution is advised, if there is underlying hypokalaemia.

- **Angiotensin-converting enzyme inhibitors (ACEIs) or angiotensin receptor blockers (ARBs)**: Since SARS-CoV-2 utilizes ACE2 receptor for entry into host cells, controversies have come regarding the use of ACEIs or ARBs. These drugs are known to upregulate the ACE2 expression. This can theoretically enhance the viral entry into cells. SARS-CoV-2 after infection causes downregulation of ACE2 and this is proposed as one of the major mechanisms behind the development of ARDS. ACE2 is known to protect the lungs from devastating infectious and non-infectious stimuli.[18] Hence, stopping ACEIs/ARBs is not justified at present. Various trials are ongoing to assess the effects of ACEIs/ARBs on COVID-19 mortality.

- **Corticosteroids**: Corticosteroids are not recommended by WHO as they increase secondary infections, delay viral clearance, and enhance mortality. Their use is restricted to a subset of patients with increased inflammation or cytokine storm.

Ageing associated decline in renal and liver function can result in increased exposure to drugs in circulation. Also, polypharmacy is common in geriatric patients. Clinically relevant drug interactions are mentioned in **Table 12.1**.[19]

Table 12.1: Relevant drug interactions of COVID-19 therapies

Drug interactions		Pharmacological effect
CQ/HCQ	Verapamil/diltiazem	↑ CQ/HCQ concentration
CQ/HCQ	Digoxin	↑ Digoxin concentration
CQ/HCQ	TCAs/SSRIs	↑ TCA/SSRI concentration
CQ/HCQ	Azithromycin/ciprofloxacin/ levofloxacin	↑ CQ/HCQ concentration Risk of ↑ QT and VT
CQ/HCQ	Metoprolol	↑ Metoprolol concentration
CQ/HCQ	Ritonavir/lopinavir(R/L)	↑ CQ/HCQ ↑ R/L concentration
CQ/HCQ	Diuretics	Risk of ↑ QT
Ritonavir/lopinavir	Statins (atorvastatin, simvastatin)	↑ Statin concentration

PSYCHOSOCIAL AND OTHER ISSUES IN THE ELDERLY IN THE SETTING OF COVID-19 PANDEMIC

The initiation of one of the most stringent lockdowns in the world has had an impact on curtailing COVID-19 in India but some deleterious effects on the elderly have been a natural result of the lockdown. In general, the Indian social milieu is unfavourable for the elderly. Although, the prevalence of the joint family system and a rural lifestyle in significant parts of the country may sometimes result in better family-based care of the elderly, the implications are not as simple. Often in poorer families, the elderly are considered a financial burden and are subject to neglect. Many rural families are also facing the modern trend of migration of earning members to urban areas in search of livelihood. In such situations, the elderly is often left to fend for themselves with meagre resources. On the other hand, although some sections of the society have modernized with both man and woman of the house involved in jobs, the elderly who stay with them are faced with a scarcity of caregiver support. This is typical to India where private caregivers and nursing homes or hospice systems have not developed yet in line with western countries. Similarly, most government-aided and private facilities which have seen a high level of technological upgradation in recent years with development of apps and online interfaces, are still not elderly friendly. Same is the case with transportation, banking, medical support services and others. The net result is that India remains, in general, an elderly-unfriendly country. The elderly in India have thus suffered from the COVID-19-induced lockdown. Caregivers have had increased financial burden; many having lost their daily income and neglect has increased. Although the central and state governments have done commendable work in making available rationed food products and medicines to households, the elderly face neglect in this too due to the complexity of the process of availing benefits. Similarly, the stoppage of public transportation has resulted in most elderly being unable to be brought for regular healthcare services which in India are still highly urban-centric. Elderly on regular dialysis and requiring regular physiotherapy due to previous stroke or orthopaedic ailments have suffered the most. Psychiatric trauma is another major issue. Many elderly patients, in the authors' practice gained respite in pre-COVID times from domestic abuse and even confinement by regularly visiting geriatric clinics just to chat with the doctor and gain solace and understanding. Many of them suffer from post-retirement depression or that resulting from spousal loss. The mental stress created on them is difficult to define. Whether all this would result in accelerated aging related complications in the post-COVID world or whether they are causing present harm is difficult to say in the absence of concrete published literature from India.

CONCLUSION

Overall, COVID-19 has been devastating for much of the world. Although the mortality statistics for India are still better, elderly have borne the brunt of the disease. Multiple physiological factors such as immunosenescence, altered cytokine response to infections and presence of comorbidities and polypharmacy result in aggravated morbidity and mortality in the elderly. Further, psychosocial effects of restrictive measures imposed due to the pandemic have also had a bearing on elderly health. The roadmap towards countering the situation and developing elderly-friendly healthcare services for the future would be a complex one.

REFERENCES

1. Wang H, Li X, Li T, et al. The genetic sequence, origin, and diagnosis of SARS-CoV-2 [published online ahead of print, 2020 Apr 24]. Eur J Clin Microbiol Infect Dis 2020;17. doi:10.1007/s10096-020-03899-4.
2. https://www.worldometers.info/coronavirus/ Accessed: 18th May 2020.
3. Chakrabarti SS, Kaur U, Banerjee A, et al. COVID-19 in India: Are biological and environmental factors helping to stem the incidence and severity? Aging Dis 2020; 11(3): 480–88.
4. http://mospi.nic.in/sites/default/files/publication_reports/ElderlyinIndia_2016.pdf Accessed 24th June 2020.
5. Wang L, He W, Yu X, et al. Coronavirus disease 2019 in elderly patients: Characteristics and prognostic factors based on 4-week follow-up. J Infect 2020;80(6):63945. doi: 10.1016/j.jinf.2020.03.019.
6. Onder G, Rezza G, Brusaferro S. Case-Fatality Rate and Characteristics of Patients Dying in Relation to COVID-19 in Italy [published online ahead of print, 2020 Mar 23]. JAMA 2020; 10.1001/jama.2020.4683.
7. Aw D, Silva AB, Palmer DB. Immunosenescence: Emerging challenges for an ageing population. Immunology 2007; 120(4):435446. doi:10.1111/j.1365-2567.2007.02555. x.
8. Ginaldi L, Loreto MF, Corsi MP, Modesti M, De Martinis M. Immunosenescence and infectious diseases. Microbes Infect 2001; 3(10):85157. doi:10.1016/s1286-4579(01)01443-5.
9. Fülöp T Jr, Wagner JR, Khalil A, Weber J, Trottier L, Payette H. Relationship between the response to influenza vaccination and the nutritional status in institutionalized elderly subjects. J Gerontol A Biol Sci Med Sci 1999; 54(2):M59M64. doi:10.1093/gerona/54.2.m59

10. Clark IA, Alleva LM, Budd AC, Cowden WB. Understanding the role of inflammatory cytokines in malaria and related diseases. Travel Med Infect Dis 2008; 6(1–2):6781.

11. Andreakos E, Tsiodras S. COVID-19: Lambda interferon against viral load and hyperinflammation [published online ahead of print, 2020 Apr 25]. EMBO Mol Med 2020; 10.15252/emmm.202012465.

12. Kido H, Takahashi E, Kimoto T. Role of host trypsin-type serine proteases and influenza virus-cytokine-trypsin cycle in influenza viral pathogenesis. Pathogenesis-based therapeutic options. Biochimie 2019; 166:20313.

13. Patricio P, Paiva JA, Borrego LM. Immune Response in Bacterial and Candida Sepsis. Eur J Microbiol Immunol (Bp) 2019; 9(4):10513.

14. Richardson S, Hirsch JS, Narasimhan M, et al. Presenting Characteristics, Comorbidities, and Outcomes Among 5700 Patients Hospitalized With COVID-19 in the New York City Area. JAMA. Published online April 22, 2020. doi:10.1001/jama.2020.6775.

15. Guan WJ, Liang WH, Zhao Y, et al. Comorbidity and its impact on 1590 patients with COVID-19 in China: A nationwide analysis. Eur Respir J 2020; 55(5):2000547. doi:10.1183/13993003.00547–2020.

16. Cao B, Wang Y, Wen D, et al. A Trial of Lopinavir-Ritonavir in Adults Hospitalized with Severe Covid-19. N Engl J Med 2020 May 7;382(19):1787-99.

17. Wang Y, Zhang D, Du G, et al. Remdesivir in adults with severe COVID-19: a randomized, double-blind, placebo-controlled, multicenter trial. The Lancet 2020 Apr 29.

18. Imai Y, Kuba K, Rao S, et al. Angiotensin-converting enzyme 2 protects from severe acute lung failure. Nature 2005 Jul 7;436(7047):112–16.

19. Summary of Chloroquine and Hydroxychloroquine Drug-Drug Interactions. https://www.apsf.org/article/summary-of-chloroquine-and-hydroxychloroquine-drug-drug-interactions/ Accessed on 18/5/2020.

COVID-19 and Neurological Manifestations

Varun Kumar Singh, Rameshwar Nath Chaurasia

INTRODUCTION

Coronavirus (CoV) is a positive-sense single-stranded RNA virus, having the largest genome amongst the list of RNA viruses. It has an average diameter of 100 nm, and is spherical or oval in shape. Large spikes of viral membrane glycoproteins present on its surface. Coronavirus primarily targets the human respiratory system. It also possesses neuroinvasive potential and can spread from the respiratory tract to the central nervous system (CNS). Previous epidemics of coronaviruses were due to severe acute respiratory syndrome (SARS) in 2002 and the Middle East respiratory syndrome (MERS) in 2012. The present pandemic of coronavirus infection is coronavirus disease (COVID-19) that is caused by SARS-CoV-2. The genetic similarity between SARS-CoV-2 and SARS-CoV is 79.5%, while similarity with bat coronavirus is up to 96%.[1] The incubation period of COVID-19 infection ranges from 2 days to 2 weeks.

Clinical Features

The common symptoms of COVID-19 illness are like fever, cough, fatigue; other symptoms include headache, dizziness, myalgia, dyspnoea and haemoptysis. In severe cases, patients may develop pneumonia, acute respiratory distress syndrome, acute cardiac problems, and multiorgan dysfunction with a fatality rate of 2 to 4%.[2]

NEUROLOGICAL MANIFESTATIONS

Evidence shows that neuroinvasion and neurotropism is a common feature of human coronaviruses. From nasal infection, coronavirus enters the CNS through the olfactory bulb.[3] Most common neurological manifestation are headache, dizziness and myalgia. Typical neurological manifestations like seizures, altered sensorium, and encephalitis in coronavirus patients were also noted in different studies.[3,4] Patients with COVID-19 have been reported with sudden loss of smell or taste.[5,6] Severe COVID-19 cases may develop hypoxia, multiorgan failure, metabolic and electrolyte derangements which may lead to clinical or subclinical seizures and status epilepticus in these patients. In a study, neurological manifestations were present in 36.4% of the of COVID-19 patients.[7] In another study, 6% of total COVID-19 cases developed cerebrovascular disease.[8] In both these studies, patients with neurological manifestations were older, had severe illness and other stroke risk factors like diabetes, hypertension and dyslipidaemia. 38% of the total CVD cases died.[8]

Spectrum of Neurological Manifestations

The CNS manifestation may be a result of encephalitis, toxic encephalopathy or due to cerebrovascular disease.

- In Beijing Ditan Hospital, first case of viral encephalitis caused by a novel coronavirus (CoV) was reported. Presence of SARS-CoV-2 in the cerebrospinal fluid by genome sequencing was demonstrated.[9]

- Critical COVID-19 cases also develop systemic toxaemia, metabolic disorders, and hypoxia. This results in cerebral oedema, with no evidence of inflammation on cerebrospinal fluid analysis. This leads to reversible brain dysfunction syndrome simulating toxic encephalopathy. On autopsy, brain tissue oedema and partial neuronal degeneration in deceased patients were noted.[10]

- SARS-CoV-2 has been reported to cause cytokine storm syndromes.[11,12] Serious SARS-CoV-2 infections often show elevated D-dimer level and thrombocytopenia, which make the patients susceptible to acute cerebrovascular events.

Pathophysiology

There are various proposed pathophysiological mechanisms for neurological manifestations.[13] A few are mentioned below:

- **Direct infection** occurring via neuronal pathway. CoV can enter the brain through the olfactory tract in the early stages of infection.

- **Hypoxia:** SARS-CoV-2 may cause diffuse alveolar and interstitial inflammatory exudation and oedema. Alveolar gas exchange impairment causes hypoxaemia and anaerobic metabolism of brain cells. This will result in cerebral vasodilation, cellular and interstitial oedema, and raised intracranial pressure. The brain function gradually deteriorates leading to drowsiness and even coma.[14]

- **Immune injury**: In severe viral infection, systemic inflammatory response syndrome (SIRS) developed. In a study, elevated interleukin (IL)-6, an important cytokine, was positively correlated with the severe COVID-19 symptoms.[15]

- **Angiotensin-converting enzyme 2 (ACE2):** It is also an important target for SARS-CoV-2.[16,17] After attaching to ACE2 receptors, SARS-CoV-2 may cause abnormally elevated blood pressure and increase the risk of cerebral haemorrhage. SARS-CoV-2 spike protein 16 also interact with ACE2 expressed in the capillary endothelium, and damage the blood–brain barrier.[18]

Diagnosis

There are two modalities of confirming COVID-19 infection: Real-time reverse-transcription PCR as well as antibody tests. A confirmed COVID-19 case will be positive on real-time reverse-transcription polymerase chain reaction analysis of nasal or throat swab specimens. Serologic antibody tests detecting IgM and IgG antibody not only confirm suspected cases, but also reveal who was infected and did not know it.

Treatment

No medical therapies definitively showed improving outcomes in patients with COVID-19. Various drugs have demonstrated *in vitro* activity against the virus or efficacy in observational or small, non-randomized studies.[19] Randomized clinical trials are going on to prove the effectiveness of the following drugs.

- **Chloroquine and hydroxychloroquine**: Inhibit viral entry and endocytosis by multiple mechanisms as well as host immunomodulatory effects.
- **Arbidol:** Targets S protein/ACE2 interaction and inhibits membrane fusion of the viral envelope.
- **Camostat mesylate**: Inhibits TMPRSS2 and prevents viral cell entry.
- **Lopinavir, darunavir:** Inhibit 3-chymotrypsin-like protease
- **Ribavirin, remdesivir, favipiravir:** Inhibit RNA-dependent RNA polymerase
- **Tocilizumab, sarilumab:** Inhibit IL-6 signaling by binding to IL-6 receptor and its activation.

Chloroquine and hydroxychloroquine are used in the management of malaria as well as rheumatological diseases like systemic lupus erythematosus and rheumatoid arthritis. These block viral entry inside cells by various mechanisms like inhibiting glycosylation of host receptors, proteolytic processing, and endosomal acidification. They also attenuate cytokine production and inhibit autophagy and lysosomal activity in host cells.

Chloroquine was found to be successful in treating more than 100 COVID-19 cases with improvement in clinical and radiological findings as well as enhanced viral clearance.[20] A non-randomized study of 36 patients also reported improved virologic clearance with hydroxychloroquine as compared to placebo. Addition of azithromycin to hydroxychloroquine in 6 patients resulted in numerically superior viral clearance (100%) compared with hydroxychloroquine monotherapy (57%).[21]

However, the concerns of additive cardiotoxicity with combination therapy do not support this regimen without RCTs. They may cause serious adverse effects (<10%), including QTc prolongation, hypoglycaemia, neuropsychiatric effects, and retinopathy.[22,23]

Baseline ECG to see for underlying prolonged QTc as well as history of concomitant QT-interval prolonging medications such as azithromycin and quinolones are must before initiating therapy.

CONCLUSION

A possibility of coronavirus should be kept in a neurological patient with or without altered sensorium in this pandemic period as only respiratory symptoms are not mandatory for diagnosis. Diagnostic tests are available in the form of polymerase chain reaction and serological tests to detect the disease early. Multiple therapeutic options are underway for management of COVID-19. In near future, RCTs results may provide the most efficacious modalities for the same. Similarly, the RCTs of the role of convalescent plasma and vaccines in managing this pandemic is going on.

REFERENCES

1. Wu A, Peng Y, Huang B, Ding X, Wang X, Niu P, et al. Genome Composition and Divergence of the Novel Coronavirus (2019-nCoV) Originating in China. Cell Host Microbe 2020; 27 (3):325–28.

2. Rothan HA, Byrareddy SN. The epidemiology and pathogenesis of coronavirus disease (COVID-19) outbreak. Journal of Autoimmunity 2020:102433.

3. Bohmwald K, Galvez N, Ríos M, Kalergis AM. Neurologic alterations due to respiratory virus infections. Frontiers in Cellular Neuroscience 2018; 12:386.

4. Desforges M, Le Coupanec A, Dubeau P, et al. Human coronaviruses and other respiratory viruses: Underestimated opportunistic pathogens of the central nervous system? Viruses 2020; 12:14.

5. Giacomelli A, Pezzati L, Conti F, Bernacchia D, Siano M, Oreni L, et al. Self-reported olfactory and taste disorders in SARS-CoV-2 patients: A cross-sectional study [published online ahead of print, 2020 Mar 26]. Clin Infect Dis 2020.ciaa330.

6. Hopkins C, Kumar N. Loss of sense of smell as marker of COVID-19 infection. 2020. Retrieved from https://www.entuk.org/sites/default/files/files/Loss%20of%20sense%20of%20smell%20 as %20 marker % 20 of %20COVID.pdf

7. Mao L, Jin H, Wang M, et al. Neurologic Manifestations of Hospitalized Patients with Coronavirus Disease 2019 in Wuhan, China [published online ahead of print, 2020 Apr 10]. JAMA Neurol 2020;e201127.

8. Li Y, Wang M, Zhou Y, et al. Acute Cerebrovascular Disease Following COVID-19: A Single Center, Retrospective, Observational Study. 2020. https://papers.ssrn.com/sol3/papers.cfm?abstract_id=3550025/accessed on April 4, 2020. This article is a preprint and has not been peer-reviewed.

9. Xiang P, Xu XM, Gao LL, Wang HZ, Xiong HF, Li RH, et al. First case of 2019 novel coronavirus disease with encephalitis. China Xiv 2020.T202003.00015.

10. Xu Z, Shi L, Wang Y, Zhang J, Huang L, Zhang C, et al. Pathological findings of COVID-19 associated with acute respiratory distress syndrome [published online ahead of print, 2020 Feb 18]. Lancet Respir Med 2020.

11. Mehta P, McAuley DF, Brown M, Sanchez E, Tattersall RS, Manson JJ, COVID-19: consider cytokine storm syndromes and immunosuppression [published online ahead of print, 2020 Mar 16]. Lancet 2020;S0140-6736(20):30628–30.

12. Chen C, Zhang XR, Ju ZY, He WF, [Advances in the research of cytokine storm mechanism induced by Corona Virus Disease 2019 and the corresponding immunotherapies]. Zhonghua Shao Shang Za Zhi 2020;36 (0): E005.

13. Wu Y, Xu X, Chen Z, et al. Nervous system involvement after infection with COVID-19 and other coronaviruses [published online ahead of print, 2020 Mar 30]. Brain Behav Immun 2020; S0889-1591(20)30357–3.

14. Abdennour L, Zeghal C, Deme M, Puybasset L, Interaction brain-lungs. Ann Fr Anesth Reanim 2012;31 (6): e101–107.

15. Wan SX, Yi QJ, Fan SB, Lv JL, Zhang XX, Guo L, et al. Characteristics of lymphocyte subsets and cytokines in peripheral blood of 123 hospitalized patients with 2019 novel coronavirus pneumonia (NCP). Med Rxiv 2020.02.10.20021832.

16. Wrapp D, Wang N, Corbett KS, Goldsmith JA, Hsieh CL, Abiona O, et al. Cryo-EM structure of the 2019-nCoV spike in the prefusion conformation. Science 2020;367 (6483): 1260–63.

17. Yang P, Gu H, Zhao Z, Wang W, Cao B, Lai C, et al. Angiotensin-converting enzyme 2 (ACE2) mediates influenza H7N9 virus-induced acute lung injury. Sci Rep 2014;4: 7027.

18. Baig AM, Khaleeq A, Ali U, Syeda H. Evidence of the COVID-19 Virus Targeting the CNS: Tissue Distribution, Host-Virus Interaction, and Proposed Neurotropic Mechanisms. ACS Chem Neurosci 2020;11 (7): 995–98.

19. Sanders JM, Monogue ML, Jodlowski TZ, Cutrell JB. Pharmacologic Treatments for Coronavirus Disease 2019 (COVID-19): A Review [published online ahead of print, 2020 Apr 13]. JAMA 2020;10.1001/jama.2020.6019.

20. Gao J, Tian Z, Yang X. Breakthrough: chloroquine phosphate has shown apparent efficacy in treatment of COVID-19 associated pneumonia in clinical studies. Biosci Trends 2020; 14(1):72–73.

21. Gautret P, Lagier JC, Parola P, et al. Hydroxychloroquine and azithromycin as a treatment of COVID-19: results of an open-label non-randomized clinical trial. Int J Antimicrob Agents 2020 March 20.

22. Kalil AC. Treating COVID-19—off-label drug use, compassionate use, and randomized clinical trials during pandemics. JAMA 2020 March 24.

23. Interview with David Juurlink. Coronavirus (COVID-19) update: Chloroquine/hydroxychloroquine and azithromycin. JAMA 2020 March 24. Accessed 2020 April 3.

Surgical Procedure and Cancer Care

Satyendra K Tiwary, Mohit Mangla

INTRODUCTION

Surgical services are at stake with COVID-19 outbreak in terms of guidelines, triage, expansion and future plans. Source control with surgical intervention is usually helpful in reducing morbidity and mortality in diseases with isolated and confined sepsis points or trouble spots. Considering the unpredictable future and rapidly changing situations of COVID-19 atmosphere, surgical practices and guidelines got to be defined which are being revised in phase-wise manners globally with update of data and prevailing circumstances. Electrosurgical devices used surgical procedures resulting in generations of surgical smoke are demonstrated to contain a spread of toxic and virulent particles thought to be capable of infecting potential with inhalation during respiration a bit like papillomavirus contracted by surgical smoke exposure.[1] Significant and solid concerns are being raised about the hazards of severe acute respiratory syndrome COVID-19 dissemination in minimally invasive procedures thanks to pneumoperitoneum-associated aerosolization of particles, also as presence of the virus in blood and stool.[2]

Exceptional conditions prevailing day by day and unpredictability in outcome making us more aware to organize the hospitals and particularly surgical units to coordinate and perform complex decisions carefully in quicker and integrated manner. Surgical concerns, roadmap and tasks for working are framed in four key areas:

1. **Surgical services**
   - Triage of non-emergency surgery
   - Identification
   - Coordination
   - Clinical networks
   - Communications
   - Rotas
   - Telemedicine
   - Virtual outpatient care
2. **Extra-working in an extended scope of practice**
   - Working beyond one's regular scope of practice as a part of a team
   - Additional training and work

- Retired surgeons and trainees
- Identification of future workforce

3. **Hospice care services**
4. **Workforce safety**
   - Infection prevention
   - Earliest identification
   - Treatment
   - Ensuring surgeons' and surgical teams' well-being
   - Periodic analysis

Considering the pandemic disaster COVID-19 knocking the door, our skilled human resources and financial strengths are in danger needing reallocation, preservation and optimum minimal utility for prolonged management strategy to bridge over the crisis. Only best planned mass casualty incident response (MCI) is that the pathway for surgical team add COVID-19 era.

KEY ASPECTS IN COVID-19 SURGICAL PATIENT MANAGEMENT[3]

1. Maximum attention for each suspected or infected cases.
2. PPE essential for all frontline warrior in touch and care of the patient.
3. Transfers by shortest route in protected way with preplanned proforma.
4. Minimum intrahospital movement of infected or doubtful cases.
5. COA (COVID-operating area) must be a separate, isolated and dedicated area.
6. Operating room (OR) should be on the brink of entrance of theatre.
7. All disposable materials and minimum materials should be used.
8. Transport team and vehicle should be an equivalent during whole journey.
9. Operation theatre must be closed after entry of the patient.
10. Whole team operational (i.e. surgeon, anaesthetist, nurses, technicians) must enter the theatre during a timely, staged and planned manner to attenuate the exposure.
11. No team member should leave the OR during the surgery.
12. Air exchange cycles recommended are >25 exchanges/h.
13. All clinical and operative documentations should be done outside.
14. Disposable materials must be disposed off after each intervention.
15. All surfaces cleaned and electromedical devices disinfected.
16. PPE must be removed and disposed off out of doors the OR in dedicated doffing areas.
17. Surrounding donning/doffing areas should be sanitized the earliest after each procedure.
18. All team personnel, whenever possible, should shower after every procedure.
19. Transfer the ward/ICU must be straight without halt.

PROTOCOL IN SURGICAL COVID-19 CASES

Preparation: Basic and initial roadmap is preparation of the protocol for precaution in COVID-19 and protection in non-COVID-19 from COVID-19 infection. Infection must be limited and contained with every protocol preparation and normal population and dealing force should be protected altogether steps of the blueprint prepared.

Location: Initial workout must include marked location for designated work and work area including transfer route and OR. Area in theatre block must be on the brink of entrance and in minimum possible space utilized in order that whole block is not suffering from working. Multiple procedures are recommended to be wiped out OR closer to the doorway area in order that other space is not affected.

Taking charge of the patient: Team taking charge of the patient must remember, well trained and full precautions with PPE must be crazy minimum manpower exposure and engagement.

Transfer of the patient: Shortest possible but pre-designated route must be utilized in transfer of the patient with an equivalent team right from the beginning till the top including transfer from ward to intervention room then return back to ward. Specified and dedicated team with pre-defined vehicle must be used during transfer with all precautions and sanitation measures with safety of other possible persons with either alarm or restricted movement and entry along the trail of transfer. Driver cabin must be break away patient and any secretions either vomitus or liquid body substance must be cleaned and sanitized by sanitary and support team system working always for safety and control.

COVID operating area (COA): Minimum manpower must be utilized in COA with better utilization of resources by shift duty and multiple teams designated to figure in COVID procedures. Minimum handling and minimum instruments with minimum distance from the patient with PPE protection of whole team and containment of secretion, discharge or liquid body substance safely and sanitation measures always adopted without failure in COA. Doors must be closed during intervention and any entry must be prohibited during procedure.

Operating room preparation: Staff must be trained and tuned with minimum equipment and minimum instruments and minimum disposables with all disposables only used during any intervention. Viral load must be minimized and reduced by increasing air exchange cycle rate (>25 cycles/hour).[4] All team members (i.e. anaesthetist, surgeon, nurses, support technicians) must be available in OR timely, with getting to spend minimum time to finish the assigned task only, but they ought to not leave within the meantime before completion of the operation but once out thanks to any reason, they need to not re-enter the OR.

Personnel dressing: All operators must wear the specified PPE before meeting the infected patient. The patient's receiving personnel inside the COA filter area must perform hand hygiene and wear full PPE.

While taking care of infected patients, gloves should be changed immediately after contact with infected material (objects, surfaces, etc.) or if any damage occurs. Operator with a beard should exert special attention to the fit of the mask ensuring adequate protection.

Some procedures likely to get aerosolized particles are related to increased coronavirus transmission: Tracheal intubation, non-invasive ventilation, tracheostomy,

CPR, and manual ventilation before intubation and bronchoscopy.[5] An FFP3 mask should, therefore, be worn by operators working closer to the patient during these procedures.

Given the conjunctiva's susceptibility to viral transmission, it is important to wear visors or goggles to guard the eyes from potential exposure of viral particles.

Anaesthesiologic consideration: Proper planning about anaesthetic protocol is essential with infected or doubtful cases during surgery. Regional anaesthesia more preferred one as compared to intubation but aggressive and planned ventilation have an edge over non-invasive ventilation (CPAP or BiPAP) procedures to lessen the risk of transmission.

Intraoperative management: No movement inside operating room during surgery should be the golden rule with door closure at the onset and opening once procedure over. Adequate and minimum manpower and consumable as well as instruments should be utilized with proper planning in any surgical procedure. No member should enter or leave the operating room in the meantime. The start should be planned with prepared end without interruptions. Viscera resected or tissue/fluid sent for histopathology must be handled properly as till date there are no study about viral load in different body tissues.

Instructions for PPE removal: Every team member must take care of while donning, doffing and disposal with prime purpose not to get in touch with contaminant. Infected or exposed parts likely to be bearing viral load must not be touched. Outer pair of gloves are to be removed first followed by body protective suite, shoe cover, head cap should be removed in sequence. Face mask and glasses must be removed followed by inner pair of gloves. Hand disinfection should be in last and with every procedure after gloves removal.

Environmental sanitization: Proper and careful sanitation of all environment in the operative area and outside in the transfer area is must for safety concerns. PPE should be worn by sanitation worker and all fluid or excreta must be disposed with safety and properly. All reusable equipment must be taken care with cleaning, decontaminating, washing, drying, disinfecting or sterilizing as per the set protocol. Chloro-derivative disinfectant in >0.1% strength must be in contact with the surface for minimum 1 minute.[6]

Waste disposal: Containers for waste disposal should be close to the working area with proper and careful disposal of all materials and after the container has been sealed and packed to prevent spillage and risk, it should be transferred with care not to damage and all precautions with PPE at every step of waste disposal is essential.

Linen management: Best way is to use all disposable linens and disposed with care in dedicated containers with PPE protection. No linen should lie just in exposed environment either it should be disposed or sent to the laundry in sealed dedicated container for minimizing the risk.

Triage of Non-Emergency Surgery

Patients should be triaged accordingly with the severity of illness into urgent (high-risk and low-risk depending upon viral load) and emergency procedures.

- Surgical needs should be assessed by hospital and surgical team to satisfy the backlog, challenges and dealing scenario if the outbreak develops.
- Surgeon should decide the necessity of the surgery with assessment of risk of delay of surgery.
- Stratification of the danger to the surgical patient should comprise a combined assessment and comparison of the important risk of proceeding and, therefore, the real risk of delay.
- Blanket policies for triage should be avoided but rather a day by day, objective data-driven assessment with changing risk–benefit analysis must be undertaken with taking under consideration expert advice and clinical opinion.

Rationing of Services

1. All elective surgical and endoscopic cases should be postponed at the present time.
2. All non-essential hospital or office should be allowed to remain home and telework.
3. All non-urgent in-person clinic/office visits should be cancelled or postponed, unless needed to triage active symptoms or manage wound care.
4. Multidisciplinary team (MDT) meetings should be held virtually as possible and/ or limited to core team members only, including surgeon, pathologist, clinical nurse specialist, radiologist, oncologist and coordinator.

Procedural Considerations

1. It is strongly recommended, however, that consideration tend to the likelihood of viral contamination to staff during surgery either open, laparoscopic or robotic.
2. For MIS procedures, use of devices to filter released CO_2 for aerosolized particles should be strongly considered.
3. MIS of reduced length of stay and complications should be strongly considered in these patients.
4. Filtration of aerosolized particles could also be harder during open surgery.
5. There could also be enhanced risk of viral exposure to proceduralists/endoscopists from endoscopy and airway procedures.
6. When these procedures are necessary, strict use of PPE should be considered for the entire team.
7. This likely includes, at a minimum, N95 masks and face shields.

Practical Measures for Surgery

1. Consent discussion with patients must cover the danger of COVID-19 exposure and, therefore, the potential consequences.
2. If readily available and practical, surgical patients should be tested preoperatively for COVID-19.
3. If needed and possible, intubation and extubation should happen within a negative pressure room.
4. Operating rooms for presumed, suspected or confirmed COVID-19 positive patients should be appropriately filtered and ventilated and, if possible, should vary than rooms used for other emergent surgical patients.

5. Only those considered essential staff should be participating within the surgical case and unless there is an emergency, there should be no exchange of room staff.
6. All members of the OR staff should use PPE as recommended by national or world organization including the WHO or CDC.
7. Appropriate gowns and face shields should be utilized.
8. These measures should be utilized in all surgical procedures during the pandemic no matter known or suspected COVID status.
9. Electrosurgery units should be set to rock bottom possible settings for the specified effect.
10. Use of monopolar electrosurgery, ultrasonic dissectors, and advanced bipolar devices should be minimized, as these can cause particle aerosolization. [9-11]
11. If available, monopolar diathermy pencils with attached smoke evacuators should be used.
12. Surgical equipment used during procedures with COVID-19 suspected, confirmed or under investigation should be cleaned separately from other surgical equipment used.

Practical Measures for Laparoscopy

1. Incisions for ports should be as small as possible to permit for the passage of ports but not leave leakage around ports.
2. CO_2 insufflation pressure should be kept to a minimum.
3. Ultrafiltration (smoke evacuation system or filtration) should be used, if available.
4. All pneumoperitoneum should be safely evacuated via a filtration system before closure, trocar removal, specimen extraction or conversion to open.

Golden Rules for Endoscopy

1. All members within the endoscopy suite or OR should wear appropriate PPE, including gowns and face shields.
2. Since patients can present with gastrointestinal manifestations of COVID-19, all emergent endoscopic procedures performed within the current environment should be considered as high risk.
3. Since the virus has been found in multiple cells within the GI tract and everyone fluid including saliva, enteric contents, stool and blood, surgical energy sources should be minimized.
4. Endoscopic procedures that need additional insufflation of CO_2 or room air by additional sources should be avoided.
5. Endoscopic mucosal resection (EMR) and endoluminal procedures should be minimized or avoided.
6. Removal of caps on endoscopes should be avoided.

MANAGEMENT IN CANCER

The COVID pandemic has created major dilemmas for providers in all areas of healthcare delivery, including cancer centres. Investigators, government agencies and professional societies have provided initial experiences and guidance on managing the continued care of patients with cancer during pandemic period. Routine visit should be done via telephone or rescheduled, oral medications should be delivered to patient's home.

The European Society of Medical Oncology and National Health Service England have suggested a tiered approach for categorizing patients into different priorities for receiving active cancer therapy during pandemic:[7,8]

- Higher priority should be given. if patient's condition is immediately life-threatening or clinically unstable, or the intervention is expected to result in substantial overall survival gain or improvement of quality of life.
- Medium priority includes patients whose situation is non-critical but delay beyond 6 weeks could potentially impact overall outcome or the magnitude of benefit qualifies for intermediate priority.
- Low priority includes patient's condition is stable enough that services can be delayed for duration of the COVID-19 pandemic or the intervention is non-priority based on the magnitude of benefit.

Oncologist should consider changing intravenous treatment to subcutaneous or oral routes, using longer intervals between immunotherapy regimens, deferring non-urgent supportive therapy regimens, using granulocyte colony stimulating factor as primary prophylaxis, and discussing treatment breaks for patients on long-term therapy.

Radiation treatment should be prioritized for patients with rapidly proliferating tumours and those whose planned radiotherapy has already begun.

Patient with COVID-19 should be treated in the respiratory or intensive care units rather than in oncology units.

Clinical Considerations for Surgical Teams

- Surgical teams are at uniquely higher risk for viral exposure.
- Structured communication before key events.
- Adapt technique to reduce exposure.
- Assume the all patients are contaminated.
- Choose effective personal protective kit.
- "Buddy system" for donning and doffing.

SAGES (Society of American Gastrointestinal and Endoscopic Surgeons) and EAES (European Association of Endoscopic Surgeons) Recommendations Regarding Surgical Response to COVID-19 Crisis

Rationing of Services

- All elective and endoscopic cases should be postponed at current time.
- All non-essential hospital staff should be allowed to stay at home.
- All non-urgent clinic visit should be cancelled.
- Multidisciplinary meeting should be held virtually as possible.

Procedural Consideration

- Little evidence regarding the relative risk of minimally invasive surgery versus conventional open approach.[9]
- Use of devices to filter released CO_2 for aerosolized particles be strongly recommended.
- Proven benefits of MIS of reduced length of stay and complication should be strongly considered.
- Avoid advanced procedures (EMR, ESD).

Practical Measures for Surgery

- Consent discussion with patient must cover the risk of COVID-19.
- Surgical patient should be tested preoperatively, if possible.
- Operation room should be appropriately filtered.
- Intubation and extubation should be in negative pressure room.
- All staff members should wear PPE kit.
- Electrosurgery should be set to lowest possible desired effect.

Practical Measures for Laparoscopy

- Incision of ports should be as small as possible to restrict leakage.
- CO_2 insufflation pressure should be kept to a minimum.
- All pneumoperitoneum should be safely evacuated via filtration system.

The American College of Surgeons (ACS) Guidelines for Triaging Surgeries of Patients with Cancer[10,11]

ACS has also organized decision making into three phases that reflect the acuity of local COVID-19 situation:

- **Phase I—semiurgent setting (preparation phase):** A few COVID-19 patients, hospital resources not exhausted, institution still has ICU ventilator capacity and COVID-19 trajectory not in rapid escalation phase.
- **Phase II—urgent setting:** Many COVID-19 patients, ICU and ventilator capacity limited, operating room supplies limited.
- **Phase III:** Hospital resources are all routed to COVID-19 patients, no ventilator or ICU capacity, operating room supplies exhausted; patients in whom death is likely within hours of surgery is deferred.

COVID-19 has had a huge and a negative effect on cancer treatment and research. Prospective collection of data on the outcomes of patients with cancer and COVID-19 across all age ranges, tumour types and treatment modalities will enable more robust conclusion to be withdrawn and can receive the best possible care.

REFERENCES

1. Zheng MH, Boni L, Fingerhut A. Minimally Invasive Surgery and the Novel Coronavirus Outbreak: Lessons Learned in China and Italy [published online ahead of print, 2020 Mar 26]. Ann Surg 2020;10.1097/SLA.0000000000003924. doi:10.1097/SLA.0000000000003924

2. Zhang W, Du RH, Li B, et al. Molecular and serological investigation of 2019-nCoV infected patients: implication of multiple shedding routes. Emerg Microbes Infect 2020;9(1):386–89. Published 2020 Feb 17. doi:10.1080/22221751.2020.1729071

3. Coccolini F, Perrone G, Chiarugi M, et al. Surgery in COVID-19 patients: operational directives. World J Emerg Surg 2020;15(1):25. Published 2020 Apr 7. doi:10.1186/s13017-020-00307-2.

4. Wong J, Goh QY, Tan Z, et al. Preparing for a COVID-19 pandemic: A review of operating room outbreak response measures in a large tertiary hospital in Singapore [published online ahead of print, 2020 Mar 11]. Can J Anaesth 2020;1–14. doi:10.1007/s12630-020-01620-9.

5. Peng PWH, Ho PL, Hota SS. Outbreak of a new coronavirus: what anaesthetists should know. Br J Anaesth 2020;124(5):497–501. doi:10.1016/j.bja.2020.02.008.

6. van Doremalen N, Bushmaker T, Morris DH, et al. Aerosol and Surface Stability of SARS-CoV-2 as Compared with SARS-CoV-1. N Engl J Med 2020;382(16):1564–67. doi:10.1056/NEJMc2004973.

7. Information about COVID-19 on the ESMO website see https://www.esmo.org/newsroom/covid-19-and cancer.

8. NHS guidance https://www.england.nhs.ukcoronavirus/wpconten/uploads/sites/52/2020/03/specialty-guideacutetreatment-cancer-march-2020.pdf

9. Zheng MH, Boni L, Fingerhut A. Minimally invasive surgery and the novel coronavirus outbreak: Lessons learned from Italy. Annals of Surgery 2020. [Accepted for Publication].

10. For more on the information provided by ASCO see https://www.asco.org/asco-coronavirusinformation

11. COVID-19 Guidelines for Triage of Cancer Surgery Patients. ACS website. Published March 24, 2020. facs.org/covid-19/clinical-guidance/elective-case/cancer-surgery. Accessed March 27, 2020.

ENT, Eye Procedures and COVID-19

Vishwambhar Singh, Ashvanee Kumar Chaudhary,
Prashant Bhusan, Hemendra Singh, Deepak Kumar Gupta

COVID-19 as a pandemic is officially announced by Word Health Organization on 12th March 2020. It is caused by newly discovered novel coronavirus. It is an infectious disease.[1]

It is transmitted by contact with infected person by:[1]

- Droplet spread of infected person while coughing/sneezing.
- Touching infected surface like plastic, steel, cardboard, etc. and then touch his/her own face, eye, or mouth.
- Chance is more when infected person is within less than 1 meter.

Most of infected person (80%) will recover on their own and require no treatment, a few patients (<20%) may need hospital admission. Very few people who have underlying chronic illness may need admission in intensive care unit (ICU).[1]

Disease can occur in all age groups. Infection is generally mild in children. In elderly and person with pre-existing comorbidity (diabetes, heart disease, lung disease, malignancy or patient on chemotherapy) are high risk to develop serious illness.[1]

Based on the current compilation of information, it is recommended that all otolaryngologists to limit, providing patients care activities to those individuals having time-sensitive, urgent, and emergent medical conditions only.[2]

There is higher viral load in nasal cavity compared to throat, if viral particle become aerosolized, it stays in the air for at least 3 hours or more. So endoscopic examination and surgery is one of the most important concern for otolaryngologist.[3]

Powered debriders and drills are used in transnasal endoscopic nasal and skull base surgery. Saline irrigation is used to clear the operative field or for cleaning the endoscope. All of these produce aerosolize clouds of vapour including any potential infected mucosal element. Infectious microdroplets spread through OT environment, and viable virus may remain in aerosol droplet for several hours.[3] Presently otolaryngologists are being adversely affected worldwide. It can commonly present like any other viral infection of common cold, influenza, pharyngitis, etc., common to ENT clinics.[1] There is also possible loss of smell and taste associated with COVID-19, it may be under reported aspect of COVID-19.[3] Fever, sore throat, cough and shortness of breath are other common presentations.

In ENT practice, COVID-19 infection is mainly transmitted by aerosol which is produced by patient during course of disease or while any OPD or any surgical procedure done on patient.[4]

During following procedures in ENT, healthcare worker may get infected by aerosol
- **OPD procedure**[4-6]
  - Examination of aerodigestive tract (nasal cavity, oral cavity, sinuses, pharynx, larynx)
  - Nasal foreign body removal
  - Nasal packing in epistaxis
  - Indirect laryngoscopy
  - Neck abscess and neck lump examination
  - Acute tonsillitis and quinsy
  - Acute mastoiditis
  - Ear examination and microsuction of ear may provoke aerosol generation due to coughing
  - Biopsy in head neck lesions
  - Microbiological sampling.
- **Emergency operation theatre procedure**[4-6]
  - Emergency tracheostomy
  - Foreign body removal from oropharynx and oesophagus (denture, coin, battery, etc.)
  - Foreign body removal from nose (battery, etc.)
  - Nasal bone reduction
  - Intubation and extubation of tracheostomy or endotracheal tube.
- **Elective operation theatre procedure**[4,6]
  - Direct nasal examination (DNE)
  - Fiberoptic laryngoscopy (FOL)
  - Elective tracheostomy
  - Incision and drainage of peritonsillar abscess
  - Powered instrumentation in head and neck surgery
  - Endoscopic sinus surgery
  - Ear and mastoid surgery
  - Nose and oral cavity surgery.

Healthcare worker who should preferably avoid working in ENT OPD in COVID scenario[4]
- Doctor, nursing officer, paramedical, healthcare worker, etc. above the age of 65 years.
- Individuals with comorbid conditions like diabetes, heart disease, chronic liver and kidney ailments, COPD, asthma, malignancy or patient on chemotherapy.
- Pregnant doctor, nursing officer, paramedical, healthcare worker.

GENERAL INSTRUCTIONS FOR ENT OPD DOCTOR AND HEALTHCARE WORKER DURING PANDEMIC[4]

- Restrict OPD consultation.
- Detail screening by taking history and temperature measurement.
- Follow guideline as described by GOI.
- No nasal or oral examination to be done as far as possible.
- No OPD endoscopy or indirect laryngoscopy should be done.

GENERAL INSTRUCTIONS FOR OPERATION THEATRE PROCEDURE

- All elective surgeries should be postponed as the government notification. Only emergencies cases should be operated, treated as suspected corona positive cases unless proven otherwise.[4]
- A prior well-informed consent is taken with patient's relatives covering clear statement that hospital as well as healthcare providers will not be responsible for risk of COVID-19 exposure and its consequences.[4]
- All preoperative investigation for anaesthesia fitness.
- If positive COVID-19 patient, we should postponed surgery until virus is clear confirmed by repeat testing. When surgery cannot be postponed in COVID-19 patient, used full powered, air purifying respirators (PAPRs) with HEPA filter (used in China)[3] or OT with negative pressure environment located at corner of operating complex, with separate access.[4] If not available, manage with normal theatre with closed doors with turning off laminar flow (if present) during procedure.[7]

High-Risk Procedure in ENT OT[4]

- Any surgery that involve nasal mucosal, oral, pharyngeal and pulmonary secretions, these surfaces are consider to have as high viral titer.[4]
- Use of energy devices for homeostasis and dissection like electrocautery, powered devices like drills, microdebriders, harmonic scalpel, etc.[4]

Specific Recommendations for Surgery[4]

- All procedures are done normally, with exception of staff in room to remain for duration of case, with minimizing the opening of OT door.
- Surgery should start as soon as possible with all staff in room in appropriate PPE.
- Most skilled and experience surgeon should perform the procedure.
- After completion of surgery, patient and whole team must remain in the room for 15 minutes post-aerosol generating procedure or extubation to allow for egress and 99% clearance in OT rooms.

SITE-SPECIFIC MODIFICATIONS DURING SURGERY

- **Nose, sinus and oral surgery:** Prior to cauterization, suction catheter with bone wax covering the finger hole is placed in the contralateral nostril. The second suction to direct and control the plume.[4]
- **Ear surgery:** During mastoidectomy, drilling through the mastoid creates droplets and aerosol in significant amount. So that, if virus present, it can cause risk of

infection to everyone in OT. Therefore, mastoidectomy is considered as high-risk surgical procedure. Any patient undergoing ear surgery should be tested for COVID-19 preoperatively, if patient is positive, surgery should be postponed until patient report is negative.[4]

- **Tracheostomy:** Performing tracheostomy on patient with suspicion or a confirmed COVID-19 patient is challenge for otolaryngologist and healthcare providers.[4,8]
- In general, tracheostomy should be avoided or delayed (even beyond 14 days) because of high infectious risk of the procedure.[4]
- It is suggested to avoid tracheostomy in COVID-19 positive in early phase because higher viral load may be present at that time.[4]
- Anaesthetist should provide adequate sedation including paralysis to eliminate the risk of coughing during the procedure. Ventilation should be paused at the end of expiration when trachea is entered and at any time when ventilation circuit is disconnected.[4,7]
- Surgeon should choose non-fenestrated cuffed tracheostomy tube of smaller size to make tracheostomy hole smaller. Keep the cuff inflated to limit the spread of virus through the upper airway.[4,7,8]
- Consider use of surgical suture rather than diathermy to prevent vapour plumes containing viral particle.[7,8]
- Suction from tracheostomy tube is done by using a closed suction system with viral filter, check periodic cuff pressures, cuff should not be deflated without considering risk to patient, staff and surrounding.[7]
- Heat and moisture exchanger should be placed on tracheostomy tube to decrease the shedding of virus.[8]
- Delay first tube change to 7–10 days, cuffed non-fenestrated tracheostomy tube to be used until the patient is confirmed COVID-19 negative. Subsequent planned tracheostomy tube change at 30 days intervals.[7]
- If patient is COVID-19 test negative, and to be moved to general ward then consider trial of cuff deflation.[7]

    In idiopathic facial paresis/palsy, sudden onset sensorineural hearing loss or, Meniere's disease high dose oral steroid is not recommended as in case of COVID-19 positive individual it may worsen the outcome. Intratympanic steroid may be given after taking consent.

SAMPLE COLLECTION IN A SUSPECTED COVID-19 PATIENT

Sample is taken by using swab with a synthetic tip and plastic shaft. Swab specimen collection vials contain 1–3 ml of viral transport medium, which contains protein stabilizer, antibiotics, and buffer solution.[9]

Sample is taken from:[9]
- Throat and nasal swab
- Nasopharyngeal swab
- Endotracheal aspirate or bronchoalveolar lavage (BAL)

    Trained healthcare professionals (HCP) will have to wear proper PPE with latex free purple nitrate gloves, during collection of patient sample.

HCP should maintain proper infection control during sample collection. No entry of visitors or attendants during sample collection. Requisition form should be filled completely and dispose all waste properly.

Respiratory Specimen Collection Methods[10]

Lower respiratory tract: It is taken from bronchoalveolar lavage, tracheal aspirate or sputum. 2–3 ml of sample is taken in leak proof, screw-cap container with 2–3 ml of viral transport media.

Upper respiratory tract

- *Oropharyngeal swab:* Tilt the patient's head to 70° back with mouth open. Rub the swab over both tonsillar pillar and posterior oropharynx and avoid touching tongue, teeth, and gums. Place the swab immediately into sterile container containing 2–3 ml of viral transport media.

- *Combined nasal and throat swab:* Tilt the patient's head to 70° back. Rotate the swab gently, insert the swab for less than one inch into the nostril till resistance is felt at turbinates, the swab is rotated several times against nasal wall. Repeat in another nostril using same swab. Take second swab rub over both tonsillar pillar and posterior oropharynx and avoid touching tongue, teeth, and gums. Place the both swabs immediately into sterile container containing 2–3 ml of viral transport media.

- *Nasopharyngeal swab:* Tilt the patient's head to 70° back. Insert the flexible swab through the nostril through floor of nasal cavity (not upward) till resistance is felt or distance from nostril to ear of the patient (approx. 8.00 cm), then gently rub and roll the swab, wait for few seconds to absorb secretion. Place the swab immediately into sterile container containing 2–3 ml of viral transport media.

OPHTHALMOLOGICAL PRACTICE AND COVID-19

Yuen et al had reported about the clinical manifestations on ocular screening of SARS patients in 2004, they had screened 45 such patients and identified common manifestations among patients treated with high dose of corticosteroids; the only positive manifestation was a raised IOP, which persisted even after discontinuation of the treatment. Since the COVID-19 virus is similar to the SARS virus, this manifestation needs to be studied in future.[11]

On the basis of symptoms, comparisons are being made with severe acute respiratory syndrome (SARS) and Middle East respiratory syndrome (MERS), both these are coronaviruses. SARS and MERS have also been known to be transferred to surfaces and contamination enters human body by routes like nasal mucosa, ocular surfaces, oral mucosa subsequently.[12]

Transmission and Investigation

On the basis of our experience with viral pandemic like SARS and MERS, we know about how COVID-19 transmission is based largely on direct and indirect human-to-human contact.

Coronavirus (SARS-CoV) is found to be transmitted predominantly form one human to another via respiratory aerosols; this aerosol may be a direct contact through touch or by fine droplets reaching the mucous membranes in the eyes, mouth or nose. The body fluids and infectious droplets of a patient can find the eyes of a normal person as an entry point of the disease and vice versa from infected patients; respiratory viruses are possible reason for ocular complications.[13]

It has been found that all kinds of body fluids may be responsible for transmission; tears are a definite risk for SARS-CoV transmission. Hence, an exposure of naked eyes to 2019 nCoV can be a potential source of infection. Viral RNA has also been found in conjunctival scrapings, tear film, pharyngeal swabs, sputum, nasal, blood, faeces samples, bronchoalveolar lavage fluid and fibrobronchoscope brush biopsy from patients with severe illness or undergoing mechanical ventilation from infected patients, raising the possibility of transmission through the faecal/oral route.[14]

Li Wenliang, an ophthalmologist, was the first personality to identify the epidemic, he raised the initial alarms on the coronavirus, he contracted the disease and unfortunately died later, he supposed, he was contaminated by an asymptomatic glaucoma patient. The summation of these information points to asymptomatic patients as a significant source of spread.[15]

Sample swabs are collected in sterile chamber and stored in human cell media, transported to testing lab facility where RNA is extracted. Later in the laboratory rRT-PCR targets the open reading frame 1 ab gene of SARS-COV-2, the procedure has been detailed in Chapter 5: Laboratory Investigations.

Ocular Manifestation

Although CoVs related virus mainly affects the respiratory system, manifestations range from mild common cold to severe forms like limb pain, fever, vomiting and other symptoms noted with MERS and SARS.

Eyes were not commonly involved with MERS-CoV or SARS, but it has been found by polymerase chain reactions on tears and conjunctival scrapings that virus was present in such patients. Ocular signs are present in only a small percentage of patients. COVID-19 patients present with pink eye, or conjunctivitis (especially mild follicular type), including bulbar conjunctival hyperaemia, epiphora or increased secretions may be present. This is about 1 to 3% of people with all coronavirus patients.

It is pertinent to note that the human corona virus NL63 (HCoV-NL63) was first recognized in a baby who presented with conjunctivitis and bronchiolitis. It was found in a study that out of 28 paediatric patients with infection by HCoV-NL63, as many as 17% had ocular signs. Symptoms can appear as early as two days from exposure to as late as 14 days.

Treatment

At the moment, supportive therapeutic strategies are the only mainstay of treatment protocol, and prevention aimed at decreasing the transmission in the population is best weapon. The chain of transmission can be broken through aggressive isolation measures; this has led to a progressive dropping of cases in the countries involved first.

Topical antihistaminic eye drops, topical mild steroids and lubricants are safe and time-tested treatments. In severe cases, steroid drops like loteprednol 0.25% or fluorometholone 0.1% may be used with caution. Repeated washings of eyes will decrease the load of pathogen and discharge, a secondary bacterial or fungal infection should be looked at, and corneal surface should be looked after for erosions. The use of protective goggles covering the whole eye, which cling to orbital margins, cannot be over emphasized as a part of personal protective equipment (PPE) of caregivers.[16]

A simple fluorescein stain will identify a viral pattern of corneal pathology. Topical acyclovir 3% has been successfully used in SARS hence may be used here too.

Precaution and Prevention

The respiratory tract is probably not the only transmission route for 2019 nCoV, polymerase chain reaction on tears and conjunctiva from patients with SARS-CoV infection have shown presence of the virus, reports suggest that about 1,700 healthcare professionals have been infected through this route resulting in 6 deaths including one ophthalmologist.

Despite being fully covered by aprons and gown as protective suit and masked respirator, health workers were still contaminated by the virus with the first warning sign being unilateral red eye or conjunctivitis, followed by development of fever a few hours later. Since the appearance of this report, healthcare professionals have been advised to use eye protection when they are in close contact with patients.

There is a controversy over what constitutes an appropriate PPE for an ophthalmologist to conduct ophthalmic examination, in context with glasses and masks. There have been instances of deaths of ophthalmologist and otolaryngologist in China and Italy, environmental virus contamination has increased awareness to favour mouth, eye and nose protection.

It is hence been made mandatory by the Centre for Disease Control and Prevention (Govt of India), for all health workers and patients to wear surgical masks to reduce asymptomatic transmission. In hotspots, hospitals require all caregivers and frontline workers to wear N95 masks.

However, because red eye or conjunctivitis is an overall common condition, and such patients more often present to eye clinics or emergency departments, it is possible that ophthalmologists are the first person to examine the patients possibly infected with COVID-19. There is always a chance of a COVID-19-infected patient having conjunctivitis to have a viral presence in his tear secretions, so the area needs to be sanitized, once the patient leaves. While performing a slit-lamp biomicroscopy, slit-lamp breath shields have been used by caregivers.

So, the dictum for all eye care providers is:
- Careful 'handwashes' after every patient.
- Avoid touching nose, mouth or face or eyes before a handwash.
- Using a tissue to wipe, if there is an urge to itch over the face area.
- Use lubricant eye drops, as dry eyes can lead to more rubbing and friction.

Despite all efforts, if there is an exposure to the eyes of the caregiver, eyes may be washed by clean running water, and soaked dry.

So, in mid of this crisis for human race the tryst continues, the human species have survived many such occurrences in history. It will definitely do this time too with a newer experience for value to basic needs of being human.

REFERENCES

1. COVID-19, Be careful, not fearful; All India Institute of Medical Sciences, New Delhi.

2. COVID19. Elective case Triage Guidelines for Surgical cares; American college of Surgeons.

3. Zara M Patel, et al. Precautions for endoscopic transnasal skull base surgery during the COVID-19 pandemic; Department of Otolaryngology—Head and Neck Surgery and Neurosurgery, Stanford University School of Medicine.

4. Advisory for safe ENT practice during COVID-19 Pandemic; The association of Otolaryngologist of India.

5. ENT UK, Aerosol-generating procedures in ENT; ENT UK at Royal College of Surgeons of England.

6. ENT UK, Nasal endoscopy and laryngoscopy examination of ENT patient; ENT UK at Royal College of Surgeons of England.

7. ENT UK, COVID-19 Tracheostomy; ENT UK at Royal College of Surgeons of England.

8. Guideline for surgical tracheostomy and tracheostomy tube change during COVOD-19 Pandemic.

9. Surface sampling of coronavirus disease (COVID-19): A practical " how to" protocol for health care and public health care and public health professionals, Word Health Organization.

10. Revised Guidelines on Clinical Management of COVID-19; Government of India, Ministry of Health Welfare, Directorate General of Health Services (EMR Division).

11. Yuen KS, et al. SARS-CoV-2 and COVID-19: The most important research questions.

12. Otter JA, Donskey C, Yezli S, et al. Transmission of SARS and MERS coronaviruses and influenza virus in healthcare settings: the possible role of dry surface contamination. J Hosp Infect 2016;92:235–50.

13. Liu J, Liao X, Qian S, et al. Community transmission of severe acute respiratory syndrome coronavirus 2, Shenzhen, China, 2020. Emerg Infect Dis 2020 doi.org/10.3201/eid2606.200239.

14. Li Q, Guan X, Wu P, et al. Early transmission dynamics in Wuhan, China, of novel coronavirus-infected pneumonia. N Eng J Med 2020; doi:10.1056/NEJMoa2001316.

15. Peterson E, Hui D, Hamer DH, et al. Li Wenliang, a face to frontline healthcare worker. The first doctor to notify the emergence of the SARs-CoV-2, (COVID 19) outbreak. Int J of Infectious diseases.2020, Vol 93, P205–7.

16. Hu K, Patel J, Patel BC. Ophthalmic Manifestations of Coronavirus (COVID19). Book, Treasure island (FL), Stat Pearls Publishing, Jan 2020.

Lockdown and Mental Health

Pankaj Kumar Gupta

PSYCHOSOCIAL ISSUE DURING LOCKDOWN

Man, by nature is a social animal. He must satisfy certain natural basic needs in order to survive. He has to enter into a relationship with his fellow men for living a life. This basic nature has probably led to evolution of family, society and nation. Why I am discussing this basic nature here is because it is getting most affected by the present lockdown announced by our government and when something is affected there is definitely a response by peoples. The intensity and direction of response is affected by people's perception towards it. If you look from my lenses, perception plays a more important role than real situations. With this background, it becomes important for us to understand what people of India feel about lockdown. A step taken by the government which is taking away their freedom, health, money and job or it is a positive step which creates a hope of coming out of uncertainty as a winner. The present lockdown is a stressful situation for people having both kinds of perception. The people feel uneasy, less sleepy, depressed and agitated in stressful situations. These emotions are more intense in people who have been quarantined due to possible COVID-19 exposure. The continuous media coverage of COVID-19 is also raising their stress level. Roy et al in their study found that continuous discussion of COVID-19 pandemic in news channels and print media make 46% of participants worried despite having adequate awareness about coronavirus infection.[1] This rising stress level is not good for people having poor coping skills. They are getting indulge in drinking excessive alcohol and some start abusing others to get out of their frustration. Even a few have started defying the order of the government. These reactions have increased the difficulty for our COVID fighters who have been given responsibility to effectively implement lockdown, which is ours only proven tool to fight against COVID-19. A study done in China is supporting the effectiveness of social distancing and lockdown in reducing the number of new cases and mortality from COVID-19.[2] But effective implementation of lockdown in India is becoming a difficult task day by day. It is raising the stress levels of our COVID fighters. It is not good for our fight against COVID-19. There is an urgent need to address the mental health issues of the general public with more focus on people in quarantine and COVID fighters for making lockdown successful.

DETECTION OF MENTAL HEALTH ISSUE DURING LOCKDOWN

Three different approaches are needed for detection of mental health issues during lockdown.

1. **First step** should start with detection of people who are prone to get stress or probably already in stress. It is possible only when people start understanding the meaning of stress so a mass awareness campaign should be organized in print and digital media to give them an understanding of symptoms and sign related to stress. The mental health professionals should also be called by the media to discuss the issue with people. Additionally, 24 × 7 helplines should be started in governments and private hospitals at state level where people can call and discuss their problem and know where to go in case things get unmanageable. The importance of this step can be understood by looking at the finding of a few studies mentioned below.

   A survey conducted by Indian Psychiatric Society recently has found a 15–20% increase in the number of persons suffering from mental illness during COVID-19 pandemic in India.[3] Another study by Roy et al in India found sleep difficulties in 28% of people in study. More than two-thirds of participants also reported worry after seeing posts about COVID-19 pandemic in various social media platforms.[1] A data on non-virus cause of death during lockdown found that nearly 884 people died in all over India till 23rd June, 2020. Among them, 40 peoples committed suicide due to fear of contamination from virus, non-availability of alcohol and financial crunch.[4]

2. **The second step** should start with evaluation of people's mental health that is quarantined. The quarantine is the separation and restriction of movement of people who have potentially been exposed to a contagious disease to ascertain, if they become unwell, so reducing the risk of them infecting others.[5] The mental health of people put in quarantine is very fragile. They sometimes felt like a person who has spread the infection and become a threat to society and society is going to put them behind the bar like a criminal.

   A quantitative study on peoples who are put in quarantine during SARS infection has found high prevalence of general psychological symptoms in them.[6] Another study by Brook et al on peoples kept in quarantine due to corona pandemic found significant distress in form of anxiety, anger confusion and post-traumatic symptoms.[7] Currently no Pan India data on mental health issues of people put in quarantine is available. But little news is coming on suicide by a few people put in quarantine. The mental healthcare professional should be actively involved for evaluation of mental health of peoples put in quarantine. The place where no professionals are available, tools like GHQ should be used regularly to check mental status.

   The healthcare professionals involved in detection and management of cases are also under severe stress. It is because of the possibility of getting infected by COVID-19 and long working hours during pandemic. A prior study on hospital staff that might have come into contact with SARS found that staffs were more likely to report exhaustion, detachment from others, anxiety when dealing with febrile patients, irritability, insomnia, poor concentration and indecisiveness, deteriorating work performance, and reluctance to work or consideration of resignation.[8]

TREATMENT OF MENTAL HEALTH ISSUES DURING LOCKDOWN

By acknowledging, recognizing and acting on mental distress during lockdown, we can reduce the impact of them on people. We have already discussed the ways of acknowledging and recognizing the mental distress. The present discussion will focus on our actions to reduce them. The WHO as well as Ministry of Health and Family Welfare India has released certain advisory for managing the mental health issues during lockdown. Many pioneer institutes of mental healthcare in India are also releasing advisory for their patients. All of them focus on three major areas:

1. *Preventing the development of any symptom in general population:* We have already discussed the role of media reports in raising the stress level of the public. So, they should minimize the reading or listening of news about COVID-19. They should believe in information given by WHO or Government of India website. It will minimize their fears. The management of negative emotions during lockdown is also an important step for preventing the development of psychiatry symptoms. These negative emotions develop due to feeling of social isolation. This feeling of isolation can be managed by a daily schedule that includes physical exercise, interaction with family and spending time in their area of interest.[9]

2. *Managing minor symptoms developed in vulnerable population:* These people develop symptoms due to negative thinking, which is a result of lethargic lifestyle. They should try to stay close to their normal routine. The person who gets stuck between excessive negative thoughts should use the power of realistic thinking. This means assessing the possibility of their fear becoming a truth. In addition to it, they can also listen to music, read books, and watch an entertaining television program in order to distract themselves from negative emotions.[10]

3. *Managing symptoms in mentally ill patients:* It is the most difficult task because these patients are already on treatment and not able to consult their doctor due to lockdown. The non-availability of psychiatric medicine near their village is also a major problem for them. So, there is a high probability of these patients coming to their doctors with relapse of illness, after lockdown is over. The telemedicine service started by many hospitals providing mental health services is an effort to help their patients but it is not enough to solve the problems faced by mentally ill patients.

REFERENCES

1. Roy D, Tripathy S, Kar SK, Sharma N, Verma SK, Kaushal V. Study of knowledge, attitude, anxiety and perceived mental healthcare need in Indian population during COVID-19 pandemic. Asian J Psychiatr 2020 Jun; 51: 102083.
2. Medeiros de Figueiredo A, Daponte Codina A, Moreira Marculino Figueiredo DC, Saez M, Cabrera León A. Impact of lockdown on COVID-19 incidence and mortality in China: An interrupted time series study. Bull World Health Organ. E-pub: 6 April 2020. URL https://www.who.int/bulletin/online_first/20-256701.pdf
3. IPS. 2020. Mental Health Survey on Psycho-social IPSYCHOSOCIAL ISSUE DURING LOCKDOWN mpact of Lock-down due to COVID-19 Pandemic URL https://indianpsychiatricsociety.org/ips-mental-health-survey-on-psychosocial-impact-of-lock-down-due-to-covid-19-pandemic/
4. Thejesh GN. Non Virus Deaths URL https://thejeshgn.com/projects/COVID-19-india/non-virus-deaths/

5. Centers for Disease Control and Prevention. 2017. Quarantine and Isolation URL https://www.cdc.gov/quarantine/historyquarantine.html

6. Mihashi M, Otsubo Y, Yinjuan X, Nagatomi K, Hoshiko M, Ishitake T. Predictive factors of psychological disorder development during recovery following SARS outbreak. Health Psychol 2009; 28: 91–100.

7. Brooks SK, Webster RK, Smith LE, Woodland L, Wessely S, Greenberg N, Rubin GJ. The psychological impact of quarantine and how to reduce it: Rapid review of the evidence. Lancet 2020 March 14-20; 395(10227): 912–20.

8. Bai Y, Lin CC, Lin CY, Chen JY, Chue CM, Chou P. Survey of stress reactions among health care workers involved with the SARS outbreak. Psychiatr Serv 2004; 55: 1055–57. MOHFW. Govt. of India, 2020.

9. MOHFW. Govt. of India, 2020. Minding our mind during COVID-19 URL https://www.mohfw.gov.in/pdf/MindingourmindsduringCoronaeditedat.pdf

10. WHO. 2020. Mental health and psychosocial considerations during the COVID-19 outbreak URL https://www.who.int/publications-detail/mental-health-and-psycho social considerations-during-the-covid-19-outbreak

Future Prospects

Kumar Sarvottam, Samir Kumar Singh, Raghunath S More, SP Mishra, Tulika Dey

COVID-19 has shaken the lives of everyone, but the crisis will be overcome. However, economic, political and social changes are unavoidable. For this reason, it is important to anticipate the world after coronavirus to ease the recovery. The COVID-19 outbreak will also have, once again, proven the need for preparing for various scenarios. Plans anticipating pandemics, or other changes, are not drawn up in vain, even though at the moment of their making that may be the prevailing feeling. The world is a dynamic place; it necessitates foresight and future preparedness. Culture of preparedness refers to a conscious and planned effort by the government to help various local resources which enable the residents to be prepared to withstand shocks also in situations in which government help is not immediately available. Culture of preparedness includes both the local capacities and networks, as well as a sense of urgency about maintaining them. The world after COVID-19 is full of uncertainty but it does not mean that we cannot prepare for what is ahead. Many opportunities are ahead of us—this is the time to vision, plan and take action.

NUTRITIONAL AND ENVIRONMENTAL CONCERNS DURING COVID-19

COVID-19, a pandemic has caused countries to follow lockdown and at many places, curfew-like situation also has been observed. Preventive measures are being taken primarily focuses on personal hygiene and protective masks or clothing and nutritional components boosting immunity, but there are some other important nutritional factors should also be considered. Being strictly at home might be a different experience altogether for majority of individuals. People experience boredom and want to get engaged in pleasure seeking activities, options for which is primarily watching TV, playing games or official meetings on laptop or mobile. Increased screen time is associated with relatively decreased physical activity. Overeating and unhealthy food preferences have also been associated with increased screen time.[1] This is also habitual of people to have food craving particularly carbohydrate craving[2] during boredom and many a times, the amount or calories are not monitored while eating and watching mobile or TV. These may lead to obesity and obesity-induced pathogenesis of various metabolic disorders. Reduced supply of fresh vegetables or fruits also compromises the important nutritional components like vitamins and minerals. Restricted outside activities may also lead to reduced sun exposure and in turn the reduced availability of vitamin D. Vitamin D deficiency is already highly prevalent in Indian population and has been linked in pathogenesis of obesity and related complications.[3] Vitamin D supplementation has been advocated as an important supplement during chest infections.[4] So, addition of supplements for multivitamins especially vitamin D supplementation and antioxidants may be advised during lockdown/quarantine.

There are reports of reduced pollution and greenhouse emissions due to widespread lockdown but long-term effects are still to be predicted. On the other hand, there are important concerns like increased hazardous medical waste being produced due to pandemic. Wuhan in China has reported to produce more than 200 tons waste per day. So future plan and strategy to treat this must be ready, one of the important ones appears to be reverse logistic network design (RLND) for management of medical waste, which is primarily based on reuse and recycling of waste.[5] A proper and frequent handwash with soap and water for at least 20 seconds has been advised by WHO as an important measure for protection against COVID-19.[6] On an average, around 20 litres water will be wasted per day in handwash, a family of five may consume an extra 100 litres of water per day, which is going to further worsen many areas in India which are already water deprived. So, a futuristic plan for increased need of water supply in these areas is mandatory. Another important environmental measure is forestation and minimum interference to the natural habitat of wild animals, as deforestation is found to be associated with increased occurrence and new emergence of zoonotic diseases.[7]

PSYCHOLOGICAL CHALLENGES AND FUTURISTIC PLANS TO DEAL WITH CORONAVIRUS

Introduction

The coronavirus disease 2019 (COVID-19) pandemic is having vast effects on all aspects of society. It is clear that direct and indirect psychological and social effects of the (COVID-19) pandemic could affect mental health now and in the future. COVID-19 has caused a massive global reset, economically, socially, politically, environmentally and scientifically almost every aspect.[8] The impact of this crisis can now be compared to that of the great depression, or even more than the World War II. A global recession is in full swing and even if you look optimistic way, it will cut even deeper in 2021 or more than that. It is time's need that researchers must set-up resources to understand the psychological, social, and neuroscientific effects of the COVID-19 pandemic.[9]

Psychological Challenges

COVID-19 infections can create a range of behavioural and psychological effects but commonly seen subsyndromal mental health problems.[10] Anxiety, including generalized anxiety disorder and panic attacks may lead to shortness of breath, aggressive behaviour results in non-compliance to treating personnel and treatment. Obsessive behaviour, depression and sleep disturbances are also observed. A novel term in psychiatry literature, coronophobia refers to excessive fear of being infected by coronavirus. For some cases, researchers reported intense fear of being infected as important predictors of the post-traumatic stress.[11] Medical personnel due to constant exposure to the infectious agent create apprehension of getting infected and spreading the infection to loved ones, leads to insomnia, can impair functioning.[12] It is imperative to remember that mass havoc and panic due to uncertainty of an illness can cause more damage than the virus itself.[13]

Call for Action

Certain fruitful activities must be for the well-being of society. So novel population-based study in multidisciplinary mental health science research is must. Researchers should take important action on:

1. Priority research on social, psychological, and neuroscientific aspects of this pandemic.
2. Need rigorous, peer-reviewed, ethically approved research co-developed with people with lived experience that can be translated into effective interventions.
3. Collection of high-quality data on the mental health and psychological effects of the COVID-19 pandemic across the whole population.
4. Psychological interventions to boost well-being and minimize mental health risks across society.
5. Experimental medicine studies to validate clinical biomarkers and repurpose new treatments for the potentially neurotoxic effects of the virus.

DRUG, FUTURE TREATMENT AND VACCINATION OPTIONS FOR COVID-19

Molecular Pathogenesis

The molecular mechanism involved in replication of coronavirus is interesting. With their S-protein, coronaviruses bind on cell surface molecules such as the metalloprotease amino-peptidase N viruses, which accessorily have the HE-protein, can also bind on N-acetyl neuraminic acid that serves as a co-receptor. So far, it is not clear whether the virus get into the host cell by fusion of viral and cell membrane or by receptor-mediated endocytosis in that the virus is incorporated via an endosome, which is subsequently acidified by proton pumps. In that case, the virus has to escape destruction and transport to the lysosome. Since coronaviruses have a single positive stranded RNA genome, they can directly produce their proteins and new genomes in the cytoplasm. At first, the virus synthesizes its RNA polymerase that only recognizes and produces viral RNAs. This enzyme synthesizes the minus strand using the positive strand as template. Subsequently, this negative strand senses as template to transcribe smaller subgenomic positive RNAs which are used to synthesize all other proteins. Furthermore, this negative strand serves for replication of new positive stranded RNA genomes. The protein N binds genomic RNA and the protein M is integrated into the membrane of the endoplasmic reticulum like the envelope proteins S and HE. After binding, assembled nucleocapsids with helical twisted RNA budd into the ER lumen and encased with its membrane. These viral progenies are finally transported by Golgi vesicles to the cell membrane and are exocytosed into the extracellular space.[14]

Many drugs are being tested *in vitro* and many have shown benefits in clinical trials, here we enlisted them according to the pathophysiological sequences of COVID-19.

1. *Drugs blocking viral fusion with cell membrane:* Recombinant human angiotensin-converting enzyme 2 **(APN01)** can inhibit the viral fusion with the cell membrane by blocking surface protein interaction with ACE2 receptor. Patients already on

ACE2 or received ACE inhibitor show lower mortality, reduced severity and lesser ICU admissions compared with controls. **Hydroxychloroquine** increases the endosomal pH and prevents membrane fusion and additionally it also inhibits viral replication. In studies, it has shown viral clearance in about two-thirds patients. **Umifenovir (arbidol)** is also in trial as important agent preventing viral entry.[15]

2. *Inhibition of RNA dependent RNA polymerase:* **Remdesivir** causes premature termination of viral RNA chain, clinical trials have shown it as a highly efficacious.[16] Another drug in this group under trial is **fapinavir**.

3. *Viral protease inhibitors:* **Ivermectin,** an antiparasitic, has shown to reduce viral RNA *in vivo* studies, clinical trials are underway. **Lopinavir and ritonavir** are HIV protease inhibitor which are under trial but have shown little efficacy in COVID-19 cases.[15]

4. *Inhibitors of interleukins:* A monoclonal antibody against IL-6 **siltuximab, tocilzumab** and IL-6 receptor blocker **sarilumab** are in trial.[15]

5. *Action on immune responses and inflammation:* Haematopoietic stem cell derived NK cell and recombinant interferons are under trial for treatment. Plasma containing IgG and IgM SARS-CoV-2 **(convalescent plasma)** has shown to decrease viral load significantly in many patients. In severe COVID-19, it has appeared an important rescue option.[17]

6. *Vaccine:* Development of a vaccine against a pathogen generally takes more than a year to be available for community. But current scenario related to COVID-19 compelled researchers to hasten the development of vaccine because of its higher mortality especially in United States of America and some European countries like United Kingdom, France, Italy, and Spain. Following are some vaccines which are in experimental stage:[18]

   a. **m-RNA:** Moderna/NIAID (National Institute for Allergy and Infectious Diseases)
   * Type: RNA vaccine made with m-RNA encoding the spike protein of COVID-19
   * Country: United States of America
   * Stage: In phase-1 trial with 45 subjects
   * Completion of trial: June 2020

   b. **NVX-CoV2373:** NOVAVAX
   * Purpose: To enhance immune response
   * Stage: Trial will start in mid-May 2020 with 130 adults
   * Completion of trial: July 2020
   * Result: It has produced strong immunogenicity in animal trial.

   c. **Lentiviral Minigene Vaccine (LV-SMENP):** Shenzhen Geno-Immune Medical Institute
   * Type: Engineered minigenes, encoding viral antigens
   * Purpose: To enhance T cell-mediated immunity
   * Country: China
   * Stage: Trial on 100 adults
   * Completion of trial: July 2020

d. **BCG tuberculosis vaccine:** Murdoch Children's Research Institute; UMC Utrecht
   - Purpose: To induce innate immune response
   - Countries: Australia, Netherlands and Germany

e. **INO-4800:** Inovio Pharmaceuticals; Coalition for Epidemic Preparedness Innovations (CEPI)
   - Type: DNA plasmid vaccine; patch-style electroporation device
   - Beginning of trial: April 2020
   - Completion of trial: Within 2–3 months

f. **AD5-nCov:** Cansino Biological Inc./Beijing Institute of Biotechnology
   - Type: Recombinant vaccine; vector is adenovirus
   - Country: China (Wuhan)
     Stage:
     a. Phase-1 trial has been started in March 2020 and will complete in Dec 2020.
     b. Phase-2 trial has been started in April 2020 and will complete in Jan 2021.
   - Subject: 108

g. **Ch Ad Ox1:** University of Oxford
   - Type: Recombinant vaccine; vector is chimpanzee adenovirus.
   - Country: United Kingdom
   - Stage:
     a. Phase-1 trial
     b. Phase-2 trial
   - Subject: 510
   - Completion of trial: May 2020

According to Ngozi Okonjo-Iweala (Chair, Gavi, the Vaccine Alliance), vaccines are the only solution to pandemics. On the basis of data collected from Ebola outbreak, she suggested that world should be careful for at least double the incubation period of an outbreak. That is why vaccination is the only effective measure to overcome COVID-19.

REFERENCES

1. Shang L, Wang J, OLoughlin J, et al. Screen time is associated with dietary intake in overweight Canadian children. Prev Med Rep 2015; 2: 265–69.

2. Muscogiuri G, Barrea L, Savastano S, et al. Nutritional recommendations for COVID-19 quarantine. Eur J Clin Nutr 2020. https://doi.org/10.1038/s41430-020-0635-2.

3. Aparna P, Muthathal S, Nongkynrih B, et al. Vitamin D deficiency in India. J Family Med Prim Care 2018;7(2): 324–30.

4. Hughes DA, Norton R. Vitamin-D and respiratory health. Clin Exp Immunol 2009;158: 20–25.

5. Yu H, Sun X, Solvang WD, et al. Reverse logistics network design for effective management of medical waste in epidemic outbreaks: Insights from the coronavirus disease 2019 (COVID-19) outbreak in Wuhan (China). Int J Environ Res Public Health 2020;17:1770–95.

6. World Health Organization. Corona virus disease (COVID-19) advice for the public. 2020.

7. Wolfe ND, Daszak P, Kilpatrick A, Burke DS. Bushmeat hunting, deforestation, and prediction of zoonotic disease. Emerging Infectious Diseases 2005;11(12): 1822–27.

8. https://www.futuristgerd.com/2020/03/a-crisis-is-a-terrible-thing-to-waste-how-covid-19-changed-our-world-futurist-gerd-leonhard-looks-back-from-the-near-future.

9. Holmes E, O'Connor R, Perry V, et al. Multidisciplinary research priorities for the COVID-19 pandemic: A call for action for mental health science. The Lancet Psychiatry 2020.

10. Angus Reid Institute. Half of Canadians taking extra precautions as coronavirus continues to spread around the globe. [cited 6 February 2020]. Available from: http://angusreid.org/Wp-content/uploads/2020/02/2020.02.04_Coronavirus.pdf.

11. Huang Y, Zhao N. Generalized anxiety disorder, depressive symptoms and sleep quality during COVID-19 epidemic in China: A web-based cross-sectional survey. Med Rxiv Preprint 2020.

12. Sun L, Sun Z, Wu L, et al. Prevalence and risk factors of acute post-traumatic stress symptoms during the COVID-19 outbreak in Wuhan, China. Med Rxiv Preprint 2020.

13. Xu J, Zheng Y, Wang M, et al. Predictors of symptoms of posttraumatic stress in Chinese university students during the 2009 H1N1 influenza pandemic. Med Sci Monit 2011; 17(7).

14. Li X, Geng M, Peng Y, et al. Molecular immune pathogenesis and diagnosis of COVID-19. J Pharm Anal 2020. https://doi.org/10.1016/j.jpha.2020.03.001.

15. Tu YF, Chien CS, Yarmishyan AA, et al. A review of SARS-CoV-2 and the ongoing clinical trials. Int J Mol Sci 2020;21: 2657.

16. Grein J, Ohmagari N, Shin D, et al. Compassionate use of remdesivir for patients with severe COVID-19. N Engl J Med 2020. doi: 10.1056/NEJMoa2007016.

17. Duan K, Bende L, Li C, et al. Effectiveness of convalescent plasma therapy in severe COVID-19 patients. PNAS 2020. https://doi.org/10.1073/pnas.2004168117.

18. Le TT, Andreadakis Z, Kumar A, et al. The COVID-19 vaccine development landscape. Nat Rev Drug discov 2020.doi: 10.1038/d41573-020-00073-5.

Index